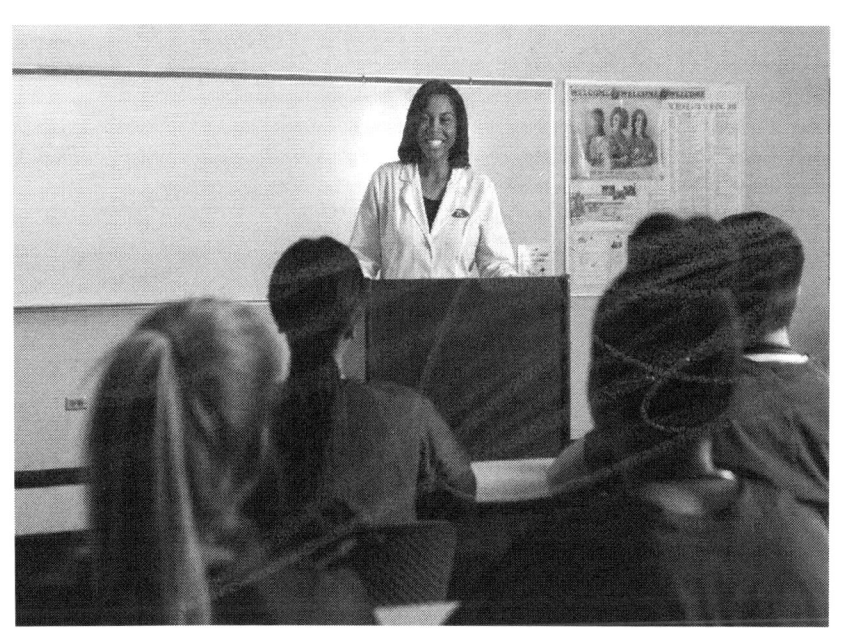

# NCLEX-VIRTUAL TRAINER

# STUDENT WORKBOOK

## for Registered ReMar Nurses.

REMAR NURSE

- a confident, well-educated individual, focused on studying core nursing content to reach their goals and place themselves in a position of leadership to bless themselves, their family, their clients, and others, specifically: as a licensed health-care professional

Regina M. Callion, MSN, RN

The ReMar Review NCLEX® Virtual Trainer Workbook

First Printing, 2019

S.M.C. Medical Media / ReMar Review

197 W. Market St., Suite #303 Warren, OH 44482

Ordering Information:

Special pricing is available for multiple student purchase orders by quantity purchases by educational institutions, not-for-profits organizations, student associations, and others. For details, contact the publisher at the address above.

Orders by U.S. & International trade bookstores and wholesalers. Please contact ReMar Review:

Tel: 1-855-625-3966

Email: Support@ReMarReview.com or,

 Visit www.ReMarNurse.com

*NCLEX, NCLEX-RN, NCLEX-PN are registered trademarks of the National Council of State Boards of Nursing, Inc. (NCSBN). NCSBN is not affiliated with ReMar Review or this educational publication.

# A MESSAGE FROM YOUR INSTRUCTOR

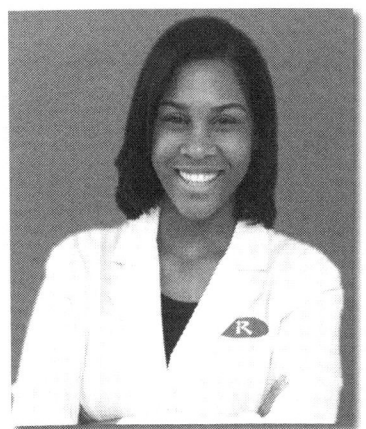

Your success in nursing will be determined by your ability to think, plan, decide, and take action. The actions you take will be based upon your core content knowledge of the fundamental practice of nursing.

These same skills are necessary as you prepare to take NCLEX®. The stronger you are with the fundamentals, the faster you will learn how to critically think and make the right decisions.

Welcome to the ReMar Nurse NCLEX Virtual Trainer the future of nursing education. My name is Regina M. Callion MSN, RN and I will be your instructor on this journey. I started my nursing career very early, at the age of 16 I was presented with the challenge to take care of my grandparents in their home.

My grandmother was a double amputee she lost her legs and vision to diabetes. My grandfather had a stroke and couldn't talk, swallow or walk. Some people might think that a teenage girl would feel helpless but I was empowered to provide care. It was the home health nurse Linda who taught me simple, straight to the point nursing information. She help me turn my challenge into an opportunity. She wasn't afraid of my age or lack of experience. She believed in me. As you begin our journey together I want to let you know that you are on the right track and I want you to see this challenge of passing NCLEX as the opportunity of a lifetime.

I need you to put pride to the side, cast away doubt, feelings of inadequacy, and any other thought that does not support this one effort here and now. I have personally beaten the odds and as a ReMar Nurse I expect you to do the same. As a company ReMar Review has helped thousands of registered nurses pass NCLEX and they are now living out their dreams. Whether this is your first time taking NCLEX or you've tested 10X or more, I want to encourage you to stay focused on this one goal – of believing in yourself! I know that you can pass NCLEX because if seen it done so many times and the only thing they needed to do was to follow the instructions, study the content, and to not give up. You are joining a global community of ReMar nurses who are committed to doing the work of passing NCLEX and getting their nursing license.

I know passing NCLEX can be difficult and I'm so glad that you decided not to do it alone. My goal is to help you study the content and make this process as simple as possible. I want to take what's in head and put it into yours. Stay focused; put FAITH over fear and continue to invest in yourself because YOU CAN, YOU WILL, and YOU MUST Pass NCLEX! Scan the code below and let's stay connected!

# HOW TO USE THE NCLEX-VT STUDENT WORKBOOK

This workbook is designed to be used in combination with the ReMar Nurse NCLEX Virtual Trainer online platform. You can also choose to sign in using your Google, Facebook, Twitter or LinkedIn account or create your own username and password by visiting your NCLEX-VT System at **ReMarNurse.LightSpeedVT.com**

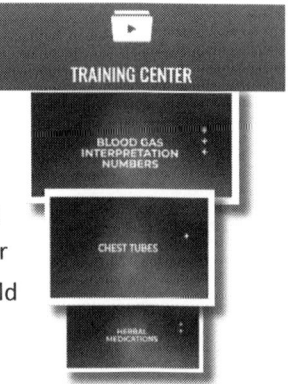

Your homepage will have many icons. Let's start with the Training Center. The training center is the first icon in the middle section of your training center homepage. In your training center you will find all of your lecture content. This is where you will also be held accountable for completing homework and practice exams.

When you click on the training center icon you will see your NCLEX information presented in multiple categories icons. Click on the select button to open up the chapters within a course. This is where you will watch your NCLEX content lectures as you fill-in the blanks to this NCLEX-VT Workbook. Be sure to use your daily study calendar to keep your training progress on track!

If you want to be an active member of the community take the time to start a discussion about the course. Your fellow ReMar Nurses may have valuable insight to share back at you as you now study together. Remember this program gives you eight-weeks of online access with renewable 30-day extensions available if you should happen to need more time with the study materials.

# HOW TO USE YOUR SIX-WEEK NCLEX STUDY CALENDAR

When you log into your NCLEX Virtual Trainer the first thing need you to do is visit the File Vault > NCLEX Resources. This is where you will find your detailed Six-week NCLEX Study Calendar.

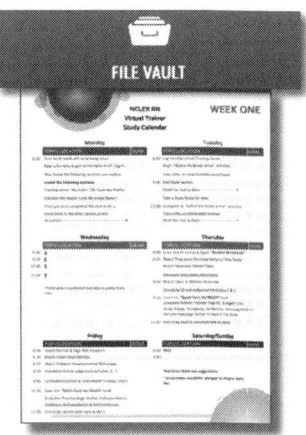

There is one calendar document for each of your six weeks of study. Simply click the link to download and then print or save each calendar document.

Please note that each day has a specified start and stopping time for your studies but don't worry these are only recommendations for you to see how much time you should be spending with your review material. Example if the calendar starts at 8:00am and the first activity takes 30-minutes to complete but you choose to begin at 6:30 am - then you can adjust that to your personal schedule but the activity should still take about 30-minutes to complete.

We recommend that your study time is limited to around 3-hrs per day maximum in order to avoid fatigue and NCLEX burnout! This is a recommendation and you may find that you are able to handle more but I want you to be kind to yourself as we go through this process together! We believe that your content should be simple, easy to understand, and straight to the point because great nurses have compassion and know their content.

# TABLE OF NCLEX STUDY CONTENTS

*Before we start I need you to do me a favor – take a moment to clear your head, steady your thoughts, say a prayer or do whatever you need to do to mark THIS moment in time.*

*I know that you have the ability to be an amazing nurse so I need you to be committed to this process of learning the content that you need to get your nursing license in the next six to eight weeks! If you're ready to go repeat after me, and say...*
*"I CAN, I WILL, I MUST, PASS NCLEX!"*

*Now lets' get started!*

*Regina M. Callion*

# PREGNANCY

**A.) Human chorionic gonadotropin(HCG) is the hormone responsible for pregnancy.**

**B.) Probable Signs**

1. Hegar's sign

2.

3. Chadwicks sign-

4.

**C.) Positive Signs**

1.

2.

3.

**D.) Naegele's Rule**

*NCLEX will give you the last date of the menstrual period.

1. add _____ days

2. subtract _____ months

3. add _____ year

*Best Calculation for months April to December

Practice Question: LMP- May 5, 2018

What is the estimated due date? _____

NCLEX Pro Tip:  If LMP falls between January to March Add 7 Days to LMP then add 9 months

# PREGNANCY

## E. Monthly Doctor's Visits and Milestone Markers

| Months | Doctor's Visits & Milestone Markers |
|---|---|
| **Up to 28 weeks** | 16 weeks - |
|  | Bi-weekly doctor visits<br><br>28 weeks - |
|  | Weekly doctor visits<br><br>36 weeks-Rapid fat production<br><br>Lightening - |

| 1. Gravidity | |
|---|---|
| 2. | |

**Critical Thinking Question: A woman has 4 children (2 singles and a set of twins) what is her parity?**

# PREGNANCY

**F. Diagnostic Procedures:**

1.

| | |
|---|---|
| **Indication** | 1. Fetal Lung maturity<br><br>2. |
| **Administration** | Invasive Procedure: |
| **Client Teaching** | 4 NCLEX Teaching Points for Registered Nurses<br><br>1.<br><br>2.<br><br>3.<br><br>4.<br><br>Watch for: |

# PREGNANCY

2.

| Indication | |
|---|---|
| Administration | Rh (D) Immune Globulin Rhogam Administration<br><br>When to give? |
| Client Education | Indirect Coombs Test |

3.

| Indication | 1.<br><br>2.<br><br>3. |
|---|---|
| Administration | Results-<br><br>Reactive is negative=<br><br>Non-reactive= |
| Client Education | |

**G. 6 Points of Client Education:**

| | |
|---|---|
| 1. Morning Sickness | |
| 2. | |
| 3. | |
| 4. Diet | |
| 5. | |
| 6. | |

**H. Danger signs in pregnancy**

1.

2.

3.

4.

If danger signs are present never assess client _____.

# COMPLICATIONS OF PREGNANCY

**1. Preterm Labor**

Medications to stop premature labor

If you Give: _____  Watch for: _____

If you Give: _____  Watch for: _____

| A.) | Less than |
|-----|-----------|
| B.) | Less than |
| C.) |  |

| | |
|---|---|
| If you give: Ritodrine | Watch for: _____ |
| If you Give: _____ | Watch for:_____ |

2. **Preeclampsia-** _____

The three defining characteristics are:

1.

2.

3.

**Risk Factors**

1.

2.

3.

4.

| ***NCLEX Maternal*** Emergency | |
|---|---|
| | |

| |
|---|
| Nursing Care for Preeclampsia: |

**Treatment:**    Only cure is to _____ the _____.

# LABOR & DELIVERY OVERVIEW

**J. Labor**

      1. Want to help labor along?

      2. When you give oxytocin when do you Stop it?

**K. Stages of Labor**

**1. First Stage**

| Stage of Labor | Description |
|---|---|
| A. Pre-Labor | Days before Labor Begins |
| B. | Cervix dilates |
| C. | Cervix dilates |
| D. | Cervix dilates |

**NCLEX Pharmacology Tips: Pain Management During Labor**

| Medication | Notes |
|---|---|
| 1. Regional Blocks | |
| 2. Hydromorphone | See Quick Facts |
| 3. Morphine | See Quick Facts |

2. Second Stage:

3. Third Stage:

4. Recovery Stage:

**NCLEX Advanced Topics:**

_____helps to tell the _____

_____

Reactive strip =

A reactive strip contains _____ _____:

A.

B.

C.  Long term variability

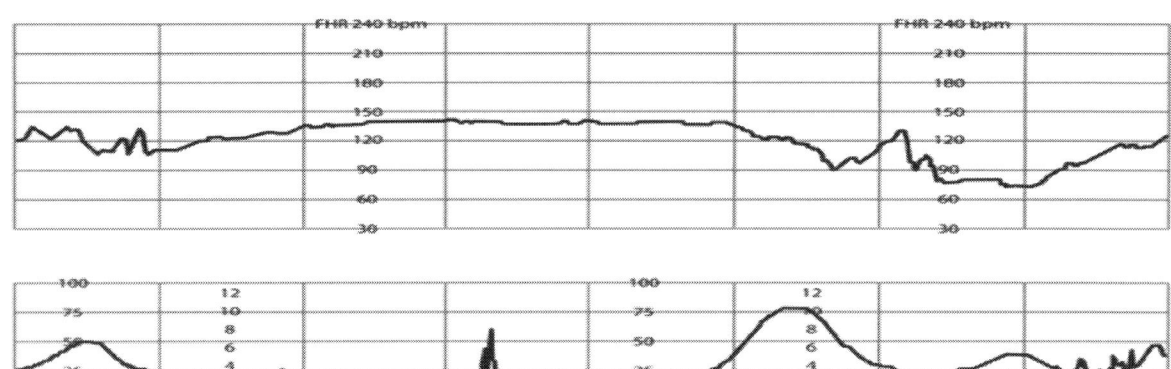

FETAL HEART STRIP ORIENTATION

Top box represents:

Bottom box describes:

# LABOR & DELIVERY OVERVIEW

## 1. Accelerations

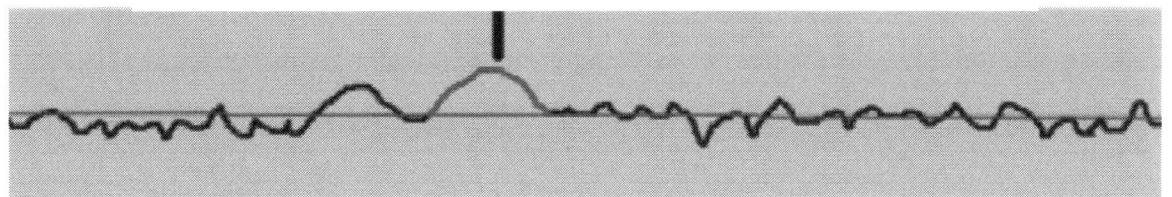

Accelerations are an _____ in the baseline heart rate.

| | |
|---|---|
| **Good sign** | |
| **Cause** | Fetal |

## 2. Decelerations

### 1. Fetal Heart Reading: Early deceleration

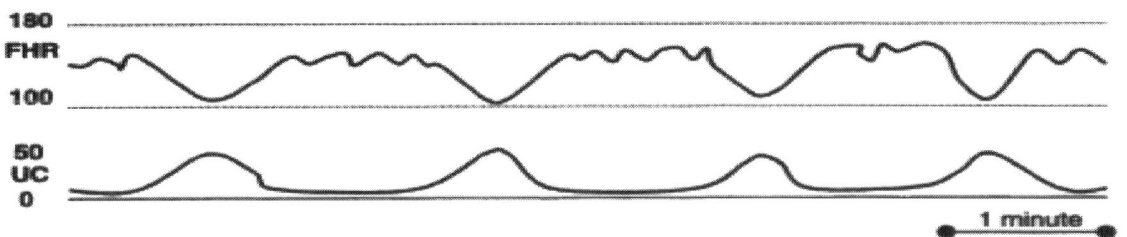

Caused by:_____

Looks like:_____

Treatment:_____

**2. Fetal Heart Reading:**

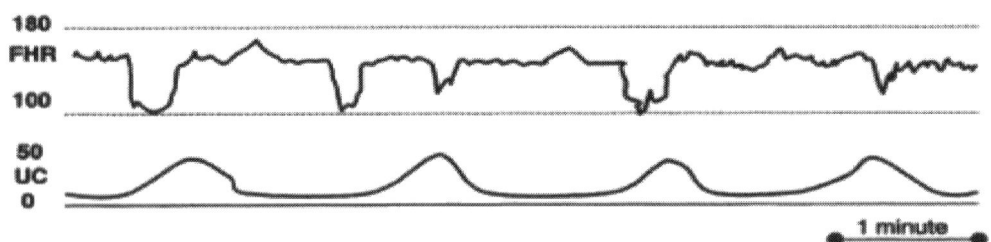

1 minute

Caused by:  Problem with the _____

Looks like: Heart rate _____

Treatment: _____

| L |
|---|
| I |
| O |
| N |

**3. Fetal Heart Reading: Variable**

1 minute

Caused by:_____

Looks like:_____

Treatment:_____

# LABOR & DELIVERY OVERVIEW

**Post-partum Assessment**

Biggest risk for post-partum complications is within:

| |
|---|
| **B** |
| **U**terus<br>Uterine atony |
| **B** |
| **B** |
| **L**<br>Color:<br>1.<br>2.<br>3. |
| **E** |
| **H** |
| **E**xtremities- assess lower extremities for edema, tenderness, varices, increased skin temperature |

# LABOR & DELIVERY OVERVIEW

| Client Education Point | |
|---|---|
| 1. | 2.<br><br>Client teaching:<br><br>1. Irregular menstrual<br><br>2. _____ gain is common.<br><br>3. Causes _____<br><br>4. Notify healthcare provider if heavy _____ starts to occur. |

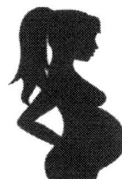

# CLINICAL JUDGEMENT ACTIVITY #1

## Match the pregnancy related word to the correct definition.

| | |
|---|---|
| 1. Lanugo _____ | A. Gravity, term births, preterm births, abortions, living children. |
| 2. HCG _____ | B. Widening of cervical os and canal. |
| 3. Abortion _____ | C. Mask of pregnancy. |
| 4. Effacement _____ | D. Presentation of fetal head at vaginal opening |
| 5. GTPAL _____ | E. Human chorionic gonadotropin. |
| 6. Eclampsia _____ | F. Pregnancy-induced hypertension |
| 7. Dilation _____ | G. Ingestion of non-nutritive substances |
| 8. Deceleration _____ | H. Shortening and thinning of cervix. |
| 9. Chloasma _____ | I. Fetal defecation in utero during labor that occurs due to stress. |
| 10. Crowning _____ | J. Stretch marks |
| 11. PIH _____ | K. Soft, downy body hair of a newborn. |
| 12. Pica _____ | L. Decrease in fetal heart rate. |
| 13. Striae _____ | M. Seizures secondary to hypertension. |
| 14. Meconium _____ | N. Spontaneous or induce termination of pregnancy. before fetus reaches viability. |
| 15. Breech _____ | O. Baby presentation is buttocks or feet first instead of head. |

Answer Box

1. K   2. E   3. N   4. H   5. A   6. M   7. B   8. L   9. C   10. D   11. F   12. G   13. J   14. I   15. O

# CLINICAL JUDGEMENT ACTIVITY #2
# FETAL HEART MONITORING

**Based on the client's current condition, choose the correct interventions.**

| Client A: Patricia Jones, 26 Female |
| --- |
| Progress Notes: Fetal heart patterns mirror contractions. Decelerations start and stop with contractions. Head compression is noted. |

1. Which intervention(s) are needed at this time? Select all that apply.

      1. Oxygen
      2. IV fluids
      3. C-section
      4. Observation
      5. Lateral position
      6. Slow oxytocin

| Client B: Shiloh Greg, 38 Female |
| --- |
| Progress Notes: Decelerations start after contraction begins, decelerations end after contraction has ended. Uteroplacental insufficiency noted. |

2. Which intervention(s) are needed at this time? Select all that apply.

      1. Oxygen
      2. IV fluids
      3. C-section
      4. Observation
      5. Lateral position
      6. Slow oxytocin

---

**Answer Box**

1. This rhythm here is early decelerations which is a normal and expected finding. Early decelerations mirror the contraction pattern. The stop and start with the contractions and are usually caused from head compression. Observation is the recommended intervention. The correct answer is 4.

2. This client is experiencing late decelerations, which is a reverse mirror image of the contractions. The late deceleration will begin after the contraction has started and will not end until after the contraction is over. The cause is uteroplacental insufficiency. The recommended treatments are: oxygen, lateral position, stop or slow oxytocin, IV fluids and possible c-section if no noted improvement.

# NORMAL & HIGH RISK NEWBORN

1.  Apgar Scoring is done at _____ and _____ minutes.

| Sign | Score = 0 | Score=1 | Score=2 |
|---|---|---|---|
| **Heart Rate** | | Below | |
| **Respirations** | | | |
| **Muscle tone** | | Some | Well |
| **Appearance (color)** | | Body normal | Body and |
| **Reflex (Irritability)** | | | |

Score at _____ minutes is more valuable.

Eyes:_____

Temperature: _____

Pulse: _____          Respirations: _____

Abdomen:_____

| Cord Care |
|---|
| Allow _____ to _____ _____. |
| By_____ cord should have _____ _____. |
| Monitor for signs |

1. _____Addicted Newborn

**Symptoms:**

What is the best way to test for illegal drugs in infants?_____

**Nursing care: Cluster Care**

**Cluster Care Examples:**

**Turn the baby on:**

**Elevating**

**Decrease**

**2. HIV Mother Interventions**

1. Use

2.

3. Can the baby stay in the mother's room?

4. Teach mother do not give

   Examples of live vaccination:

5. Can you give Vitamin K shot?

**3. Fetal**

| Characteristics to know |
| --- |
| 1. |
| 2. |
| 3. |
| 4. |
| Risk for: |
| Treatment: |

4.

Definition:

Watch for:

Treatment:

_____may be required.

Client Safety Point Position:

5.

Treatment:

Client Education for Parents:

NCLEX Tip: Nutrition is a major concern for these birth defects.

# INFANT HEART DEFECTS

| Blue Baby | Pink Baby |
|---|---|
| 1.<br><br>2.<br><br>3.<br><br>4. | 1.<br><br>2.<br><br>Hole between 2 upper chambers<br><br>3.  Patent Ductus Ateriosus- |

All Blue Baby problems begin with the letter _____.
*Emergency Position:*

Most Important Infant Heart Defect

| Tetralogy of Fallot |
|---|

| Mnemonic | Clinical Condition |
|---|---|
| R | Right Ventricular Hypertrophy |
| O |  |
| P | Pulmonary |
| V |  |

# INFANT HEART DEFECTS

How should a nurse identify a child?

**Critical Thinking Questions**

1.  An infant with Tetralogy of fallot is discharged with a prescription for digoxin elixir. The nurse should instruct the mother to:

    1.  Administer the medication using a nipple.
    2.  Administer the medication using the calibrated dropper in the bottle.
    3.  Administer the medication using a plastic baby spoon.
    4.  Administer the medication in a baby bottle with 1. Oz of water.

2.  A nurse is caring for an infant diagnosed with Tetralogy of fallot which of the following are expected findings? Select all that apply.

    1.  Clubbing of the fingers
    2.  Dyspnea with activity
    3.  Hypoglycemia
    4.  Fever
    5.  Cyanosis

3.  Calculate the Apgar Score for each category and report the total.

| Baby Jones | Score |
| --- | --- |
| Heart rate = 85 | |
| Respirations= Full and normal | |
| Muscle= No spontaneous movements noted | |
| Appearance= Arms & legs blue | |
| Reflex= No response | |
| **Total** | |

# PEDIATRIC DEVELOPMENTAL MILESTONES

| AGE | ACTIVITY | NCLEX TIPS |
|---|---|---|
| S | Erikson's Stages of Psychosocial development:<br><br>Freud Stages of Psychosexual development: | Best Toy |
| **6-9 months**<br><br>O_____<br><br>P_____ | | First Solid food?<br><br>Best Toy |

| | | |
|---|---|---|
| **9-12 months**<br>. | | Best toy: |
| **1-3 years old**<br>. | Gross Motor Skills<br><br><br>Drinks from a cup?<br>Uses a spoon?<br>Favorite word?<br><br>Erikson's Stages of Psychosocial development:<br><br><br>Freud Stages of Psychosexual development: | Which is the best option?<br><br>1. Explain<br>2. Remove a favorite object<br>3. Time Out<br>4. Spanking |

| 4-6 years old | Erikson's Stages of Psychosocial development:<br><br>Freud Stages of Psychosexual development: | |
|---|---|---|
| 7-12 years old | Erikson's Stages of Psychosocial development:<br><br>Freud Stages of Psychosexual development: | |
| 13-18 years old<br><br>**Peer Association** | Erikson's Stages of Psychosocial development:<br><br>Identity vs. Role Confusion<br>　13-21 years old<br><br>Freud Stages of Psychosexual development:<br><br>Genital<br>　12-20 years old | |

| | |
|---|---|
| **Children's Response to Death** | |
| **Infants & Toddlers**<br>**0-3 years old** | Only live in the _____.<br><br>No sense of _____.<br><br>Do not separate from _____.<br><br>Can sense sadness in _____. |
| **Preschoolers**<br>**4-6 years-old** | See death as _____.<br><br>Think it is like _____.<br><br>Reversible and _____.<br><br>Behavior may _____. |
| **School Age**<br>**7-12 years-old** | Feel _____ is a punishment.<br><br>Understands_____. |
| **Adolescents**<br>**13-18 years-old** | _____ expressed towards<br><br>Death.<br><br>Find it difficult to _____  _____.<br><br>May want to help with funeral  arrangements. |

# NCLEX PRACTICE QUESTIONS

1. A registered nurse is teaching a conference on the normal development of four-year-olds.. Which of the following statements should be included? Select all that apply.

   1. "The child may exhibit a fear of the dark"
   2. "The normal weight should double during this age."
   3. "According to Erickson's Stages of Psychosocial development the child is experiencing industry vs. inferiority.
   4. "Children at this age understand death to be permanent."

2. A teenager is admitted to the hospital with a diagnosis influenza. The teenager refuses to let his friends come to visit. The nurse should know this is a result of:

   1. His inability to explain what is happening to the friends.
   2. His perception of altered body image.
   3. His need to be in the center of attention.
   4. His anger on being left out of school activities.

3. The nurse is caring for an 11-month-old admitted to the hospital with a respiratory infection. The child is in a croup tent with supplemental oxygen. Which toy is **most** appropriate for the nurse to recommend to the parents?

   1. A push-pull toy.
   2. A toy car.
   3. A soft multi-colored ring stacking set.
   4. A wind-up jack in the box on wheels.

# CLINICAL JUDGEMENT ACTIVITY #3

**Apgar Scoring** - Calculate the correct Apgar score for each client.

## Baby A

| Indicator | Points |
|---|---|
| 1. Appearance: Pink torso and extremities | |
| 2. Pulse: 100 | |
| 3. Respirations: Irregular ventilation | |
| 4. Irritability: Coughing | |
| 5. Activity: Moving actively | |

## Baby B

| Indicator | Points |
|---|---|
| 1. Appearance: Pink torso, blue extremities | |
| 2. Pulse: 60 | |
| 3. Respirations: Strong loud cry | |
| 4. Irritability: Facial grimace | |
| 5. Activity: Flaccid | |

**Baby C**

| Indicator | Points |
|---|---|
| 1. Appearance: Blue/Pale | |
| 2. Pulse: 45 | |
| 3. Respirations: Absent | |
| 4. Irritability: Minimal response to stimulation | |
| 5. Activity: Some flexion | |

Answer Box:
Baby A: 1. 2 2. 2 3. 1 4. 2 5.2 Total = 9
Baby B: 1. 1 2. 1 3. 2 4. 1 5. 0 Total = 5
Baby C: 1. 0 2. 1 3. 0 4. 1 5. 1 Total= 3

# CLINICAL JUDGEMENT ACTIVITY #4

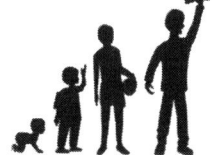

Circle the correct age based on the developmental milestones achieved.

| | | | |
|---|---|---|---|
| 1. Forms social groups, swims, skates, and uses complete sentences.<br><br>A. 15-18 months old<br><br>B. 3-4 years old<br><br>C. 10-12 years old | 2. Plays with toes, has stranger anxiety, turns onto back.<br><br>A. 2 months old<br><br>B. 12 months old<br><br>C. 6 months old | 3. Walks well, uses three word phrases, is potty- trained.<br><br>A. 15-18 months old<br><br>B. 2 years old<br><br>C. 5 years old | 4. Dresses self, catches a ball, hops on 1 foot.<br><br>A. 2 years old<br><br>B. 4 years<br><br>C. 6 years old |
| 5. Walks with assistance or alone, point sto named objects, drinks from a cup.<br><br>A. 8 months old<br><br>B. 12 months old<br><br>C. 3 years old | 6. Reflex activity noted, makes eye contact, cries to communicate.<br><br>A. 1 month old<br><br>B. 5 months old<br><br>C. 8 months old | 7. Speaks clearly, uses future tenses such as "My birthday is coming soon", prints some letters.<br><br>A. 3 years old<br><br>B. 5 years old<br><br>C. 10 years old | 8. Displays temper tantrums, says single words, points to body parts<br><br><br>A. 12 months old<br><br>B. 18 months old<br><br>C. 4 years old |

Answer Box.    1. C    2. C    3. B.    4. B.    5. B.    6. A.    7. B.    8. B

You need to do homework for this section and then begin your next section with NCLEX Activity pages along Clinical Judgement activities. Great job so far!

# CLINICAL JUDGEMENT ACTIVITY #5

1. A client is 34 weeks pregnant. Which of the following statements would make a nurse suspect preeclampsia?

> 1. "I have cravings for non-food substances."
> 2. "I no longer wear my wedding ring because it doesn't fit."
> 3. "I no longer wear my pants because they no longer fit."
> 4. "Sometimes I feel lightheaded and have to lie down."

2. A nurse is caring for a post-partum client who is interested in birth control pills as a form of contraceptive. The nurse should explain the cause of breast tenderness and possible nausea is due to which of the following?

> 1. Increased luteinizing hormone.
> 2. Increased follicle-stimulating hormone.
> 3. Increased estrogen levels.
> 4. Decreased estrogen levels.

3. A nurse is working in a wellness clinic. A client is scheduled to have a Papanicolaou smear. What are the **most** appropriate instructions for the nurse to provide?

> 1. "Do not eat anything for 8 hours before the exam."
> 2. "If you are experiencing a sexually transmitted disease please bring your partner in to be tested as well."
> 3. "If you are menstruating you will still be required to take the exam."
> 4. "Do not place anything in the vagina within 24 hours of your examination."

4. A registered nurse is instructing a group of teenage boys on the female anatomy. She should explain that fertilization normally takes place in the:

> 1. uterus
> 2. cervix
> 3. ovary
> 4. fallopian tube

5. Sperm production takes place in which of the following?

> 1. Vas deferens
> 2. Testes
> 3. Prostate
> 4. Androgens

6. A client is suspected of having placenta previa. Which of the following is a sign of the condition?

> 1. Maternal bradycardia
> 2. Prolapsed cord
> 3. Hyperglycemia
> 4. Painless bleeding

## Clinical Judgement Answers

1. 4-Clients experiencing swelling or edema in the hands, face, or around the eyes are presenting signs of preeclampsia. Clients may experience the other options as the pregnancy progresses and there is an increase of weight and hormones.

2. 3-Oral contraceptives cause an increase in estrogen levels which may result in breast tenderness.

3. 4-The best advice for the nurse to provide is not to insert anything into the vaginal canal. The Papanicolaou or Pap test is used to check for cervical cancer. The client should avoid tampons, douching, and sexual intercourse. When preparing for a Pap exam the client should not be on her menses. The client is allowed to eat normally. Sexual partners are not required to be present or be tested.

4. 4-Fertilizations takes place in the fallopian tube and then the egg will migrate to the uterus for growth. All other choices are incorrect.

5. 2-Sperm production occurs in the testes.

6. 4-Placenta previa is a medical emergency that requires immediate treatment. Normal contractions and painless bleeding is an early indication of the condition.

# MATERNAL & CHILD HEALTH PROGRESS EXAM

**Directions:**

These are your progress exam questions. Please do the items inside the book and then take the exam in your virtual trainer for a score. You will get the correct answers after each question in the virtual trainer. Mark the correct answer in this book. I have provided each exam in the workbook so that you will have the record. Once your test is complete in the virtual trainer, you will not be able to view your exam again. Mark your answers in the book. You will need 95% to pass the exam.

1. A client with severe pregnancy-induced hypertension is admitted to the maternity unit. The client asks the nurse, "Is my baby going to be ok?" The **most** appropriate response by the nurse would be?

    A. The healthcare provider will tell us precisely what is going to happen.
    B. If you follow the medical instructions, all things will be well.
    C. The baby will be fine; it is protected inside the uterus.
    D. We are going to monitor your baby while you are here constantly.

2. A nurse has just received a client who has pre-eclampsia and must remain on bed rest at home. The client starts to cry and tells the nurse that she has three children at home that need her for care. The nurse's best response should be:

    A. You'll need someone to care for the children.
    B. You do not need to worry about how you will take of them at this time.
    C. You can get a babysitter to help while your husband is at work during the day.
    D. You will still be able to fix small meals and do light activities.

3. A nurse is working in a prenatal clinic. While preparing a client for a pelvic examination, the client states, "Why must I be pregnant; this is the wrong time for me?" What is the **most** therapeutic response by the nurse?

    A. No time is ever the right time to be pregnant.
    B. Why don't you want to be pregnant?
    C. This emotion is a normal response to pregnancy
    D. You don't seem excited about the possibility of being pregnant.

4. A pregnant client with an infection tells the nurse that she has taken tetracycline for infections on other occasions and would prefer to take it now. The nurse should tell the client that tetracycline is avoided in the treatment of infections in pregnant woman. This is due to which of the following?

    A. Tetracycline can cause damage to the tooth development in the baby.
    B. Tetracyclines can reduce breastmilk.
    C. Tetracyclines can produce an allergic response to the drug.
    D. Tetracyclines can increase the baby's tolerance to the medication.

5. The physician sees a 37-year-old who is Rh-negative during the first trimester of pregnancy. The nurse's teaching is valid if the client understands that she will first receive Rho(D) immune globulin (RhIg) at:

    A. 14 weeks
    B. 28 weeks.
    C. 36 weeks
    D. 40 weeks

6. The nurse should be aware that the only anticoagulant medication that can safely be administered during pregnancy is which of the following?

    A.   Warfarin sodium
    B.   Anisindione
    C.   Heparin sodium
    D.   Dicumarol

7. A client is receiving oxytocin, and the nurse is aware of the adverse effects of this medication. The nurse should decrease the oxytocin if the following sign is present:

    A.   A fetal heart rate of 120 to 150 beats per minute.
    B.   Intrauterine pressure of 60 mm Hg
    C.   Contractions with a duration of 30 seconds.
    D.   Contractions that occur more frequently than every 2 minutes.

8. A nurse is ordered to administer terbutaline to a client in preterm labor. The nurse is aware that a side effect of this medication is:

    A.   Decreased pulse pressure
    B.   Hypokalemia
    C.   Increased uterine contractions.
    D.   Tachycardia

9. The nurse is caring for a client with pre-eclampsia who is receiving magnesium sulfate. The client is showing signs of magnesium sulfate toxicity. The nurse is aware that these signs can be reversed by administering which of the following?

    A.   Calcium gluconate
    B.   Edetate disodium
    C.   Hydralazine hydrochloride
    D.   Sodium polystyrene sulfonate

10. A nurse is caring for a client who suspects she is pregnant. A positive early diagnosis of pregnancy is based on the presence of:

    A.   Chorionic gonadotropin
    B.   Chadwick's sign
    C.   A fetal heart rate
    D.   Quickening

11. Fill in the blank to make the sentence correct.

The nurse caring for a child with AIDS should use _____ isolation precautions.

12. The nursing diagnosis with the highest priority for a child diagnosed with AIDS would be:

    A.   High risk for bleeding.
    B.   High risk for injury.
    C.   High risk for pain.
    D.   High risk for infection.

13. After the repair of a cleft lip, the nurse will provide nutrition for the baby via:

    A. A plastic teaspoon
    B. A straw
    C. A rubber-tipped syringe
    D. Nasogastric tube feedings

14. A nurse is caring for a child who recently returned from surgery. Following a tonsillectomy, the first fluid the nurse should give the 10-year-old child is:

    A. Ice water
    B. Ice cream
    C. Warm milk
    D. Orange juice

15. The nurse is caring for an infant with tetralogy of Fallot, and there are signs of decreased oxygenation. The nurse is aware the goal of surgery to treat tetralogy of Fallot is to increase the blood flow to the directly:

    A. Brain
    B. Lungs
    C. Right ventricle
    D. Myocardium

# AGE SPECIFIC NURSING CARE

No matter the age all clients have the same rights for:

    1.

    2. Privacy

    3.

    4.

    5.

    6.

    7. Involvement of family and/or significant others.

| Age Group 1-12 |
|---|

The top 2 nursing concerns are:

1.

Pediatric patients are 3 times more likely to have a medication error.

2.

Before administering a medication ask client for:

| **Critical Thinking Question:** If a patient is too young, can the parents answer? _____ |
|---|

**NCLEX Teaching Point:**

Patients have to be positioned properly before giving medications or feedings to prevent

_____.

Separation from the primary care giver is:

Adults number one fear is:

| ReMar Tip: |
| --- |
|  |

| Age Group: 13-18 |
| --- |

Goals:

· Develop _____with the opposite _____.

· Establishing a _____ _____.

· Coping with _____ _____.

They have the need to establish independence from primary care giver.

| Medication | NCLEX Points |
| --- | --- |
|  | 1. Elevate the |
|  | 2. Use |
|  | 3. Do not take with vitamin |
|  | 4. Can cause inflammation of |

**Psych Priority:**

1.

<table>
<tr><td align="center">**Age Group: 19-40**</td></tr>
</table>

1. Resolve _____
2. When sick rearranging responsibilities of work, child rearing etc.

<table>
<tr><td align="center">**Age Group: 40-60**</td></tr>
</table>

#1 Concern is to:

<table>
<tr><td align="center">**Community Health Nursing**</td></tr>
</table>

**There are 3 levels of prevention:**

| Level of Prevention | Techniques |
|---|---|
| **1. Primary Prevention**<br><br>**The Goal: Keep healthy people healthy.** | |
| **2. Secondary Prevention**<br><br>**The Focus: early recognition &** | |
| **Tertiary Prevention**<br><br>**The Focus: contain damage of an illness and** | |

# AGE SPECIFIC NURSING CARE

**Psych concerns:**

Caring for _____ & _____ at the same time.

| Age Group 60-and over |
|:---:|

**Goals**

Positively _____ the loss of a _____.

Transition into _____.

Maintain physical _____ and prevent cognitive _____.

### NCLEX Nursing concerns

| | |
|---|---|
| 1. | Lower metabolism<br>Higher body fat<br><br>Check for:<br><br>Assess client's: |
| 2. | Prevention of Falls<br><br>1.<br><br>2.<br><br>3.<br><br>#1 thing to give:<br><br>Non slip socks, call light in reach, bowel/bladder program where you are able to anticipate ambulation needs |
| 3. | 1.<br><br>What is the most important lab value to determine the nutritional status of a client?<br><br>2.<br><br><br>3. |

# EXPECTED CHANGES DURING AGING

| System | Changes Tested on NCLEX |
|---|---|
| 1. | Decreased _____ output<br><br>Increase:<br><br>Peripheral circulation: |
| 2. | Increased<br><br>Decreased<br><br>Is it normal to wear oxygen? |
| 3. | Decline in the ability to: |
| 4. Reproductive System | Women decrease:<br><br>Men decrease:<br><br>Sexual Changes<br><br>Women:<br><br>Men: |

| | |
|---|---|
| **5.** | Decreased range<br><br>Decreased _____ _____.<br><br>Decreased in overall<br><br>Bone loss |
| **6.** | Kidneys-<br><br>Bladder-<br><br>Dehydration is a common issue<br><br>Is urinary incontinence normal?<br><br>Kegel exercises- |
| **Gastrointestinal System** | _____mouth<br><br>Constipation<br><br>Delayed gastric emptying<br><br>_____ability decreases<br><br>Is tooth loss a normal part of aging? |

| | |
|---|---|
| **Nervous System** | Decreased activity in CNS & PNS<br><br>Decrease in _____ time and reflex times.<br><br> Mental function should<br><br>_____   _____.<br><br>If intelligence decreases a disease process is present. |
| **Immune System** | _____ in the _____of immune system.<br><br><br>Encourage: |
| **Endocrine System** | Decrease secretion of:<br><br><br>Decrease in:<br><br>Will a decreased insulin production   make the blood sugar increased or decreased? |
| **Sensory System** | Loss of: |

# CLINICAL JUDGEMENT ACTIVITY #6

Consider each scenario and choose the correct answer related to the care of the older adult client.

1. Which of the following are normal respiratory changes associated with advanced age? Select all that apply.

    1. Changes in the anteroposterior diameter of the chest
    2. Loss of elastic tissue surrounding the alveoli.
    3. Decreased residual volume.
    4. Increased risk of lung cancer.
    5. Dietary carbohydrate levels decrease.

2. The bone changes associated with aging frequently result from a loss of:

    1. osteoporosis
    2. calcium
    3. vitamin C
    4. folate

3. The study of the process of aging is called:

    1. Geriatrics
    2. Ageism
    3. Gerontology
    4. Anthropology

---

Answer box

1. 1, 2, The client with advanced age will experience changes in the anteroposterior diameter of the chest as the overall diameter of the thoracic cage decreases and a rounding of the thoracic spine occurs. Age related loss of lung elastic recoil will cause a loss also of alveolar surface area. The other options are not associated with advanced maternal age.

2. The correct answer is 2. The loss of calcium affects bone changes seen with aging.

3. The study of the process of aging is called gerontology. The ending –logy indicates the study of a subject. Geriatrics is the branch of medication dealing with the health and care of old people. Ageism is the prejudice or discrimination based on a person's age. Anthropology is the study of the human societies and their cultures.

---

# PHYSIOLOGICAL CHANGES HOMEWORK EXAM

Directions:

These are your homework questions. Please do the items inside the book and enter your answers in your virtual trainer for a score. Once your test is complete, you will not be able to view your exam again. Mark your answers in the book. You will need an 95% to pass the exam.

**1. Number Erikson's Stages of Psychosocial Development according to age.**

| | |
|---|---|
| | **Generativity vs. Stagnation** |
| | **Industry vs. Inferiority** |
| | **Ego Integrity vs. Despair** |
| | **Autonomy vs. Shame & Doubt** |
| | **Identity vs. Role Confusion** |
| | **Trust vs. Mistrust** |
| | **Initiative vs. Guilt** |
| | **Intimacy vs. Isolation** |

**2. According to Erikson's Stages of Psychosocial Development, match the approximate age to the psychosocial crisis.**

| | |
|---|---|
| 1. Infant -18 months | Ego Integrity vs. Despair |
| 2. 18 months -3 years old | Intimacy vs. Isolation |
| 3. 3-5 years old | Trust vs. Mistrust |
| 4. 5-13 years old | Industry vs. Inferiority |
| 5. 13-21 years old | Generativity vs. Stagnation |
| 6. 21-39 years old | Identity vs. Role Confusion |
| 7. 40-65 years old | Initiative vs. Guilt |
| 8. 65 and older | Autonomy vs. Shame & Doubt |

3. Which of the following is not a way that HIV can be transmitted?

    A.  Sharing needles
    B.  Breastfeeding
    C.  Saliva
    D.  Semen
    E.  Pre-seminal fluids

4. A nurse is caring for a child who was potentially exposed to alcohol as a fetus. Which physical feature is associated with fetal alcohol syndrome?

    A.  Smaller than an average brain
    B.  Decreased activity
    C.  Poor vision
    D.  Larger physical stature

5. When assessing the newborn infant, what is the tendency of an infant to reach with his or her mouth when touched there?

    A.  Rooting reflex
    B.  Startling reflex
    C.  Sucking reflex
    D.  Refeeding reflex

6. Which of the following assessment findings would the nurse expect to find in a newborn addicted to cocaine?

    A.  Sleepiness
    B.  Irritable
    C.  Lethargy
    D.  Willingness to cuddle

7. A registered nurse is caring for a six weeks old newborn who has had a cleft lip repair 6 hours ago. Which nursing intervention is appropriate when caring for this child's surgical incision?

    A.  Rinse the incision with sterile water after feeding.
    B.  Clean the incision only when serous exudate forms.
    C.  Rub the incision gently with a sterile cotton-tipped swab.
    D.  Replace the Logan bar carefully after cleaning the incision.

8. A nurse is caring for a 21-year-old female client with reported abdominal pain. The client states she is six weeks pregnant. Which finding indicates a possible ectopic pregnancy?

    A.  Vaginal bleeding
    B.  Stabbing pain in the lower quadrant
    C.  Abdominal cramping
    D.  Stabbing pain in the upper quadrant

9. A nurse is caring for a 39-weeks pregnant client. The client comes into the labor & delivery unit with regular contractions. Which of the following complications should the nurse suspect when the client informs her that she has placenta previa?

    A.   Fever
    B.   Vomiting
    C.   Vaginal bleeding
    D.   The abrupt flow of vaginal fluids

10. A nurse is teaching a prenatal class at the community health clinic. Which of the following should not be included as a factor of breast changes during pregnancy?

    A.   Areolas will darken.
    B.   Nipples become more erect.
    C.   Colostrum may leak before delivery.
    D.   Nodules will begin to form inside the breast tissue.

11. A nurse is caring for a newborn infant of a diabetic mother. Which finding in the newborn would require immediate action by the nurse?

    A.   Jitteriness
    B.   Crying
    C.   Yawning
    D.   Reaching

12. A nurse is caring for a pregnant client in active labor. The nurse is preparing the client for a vaginal delivery and notices a papular lesion on the perineum. Which is the initial action of the nurse?

    A.   Prepare the client for a C-section.
    B.   That is not correct.
    C.   Document the finding.
    D.   Notify the healthcare provider.

13. A nurse is caring for a pregnant client who is eight weeks pregnant. The client presents with increased softening of the cervix. The nurse is aware this is called which of the following?

    A.   Goodell's sign
    B.   Godwin's sign
    C.   Chadwick's sign
    D.   Ballottment
    E.   Montgomery's sign
    F.   Vascular hyperplasia

14. The healthcare provider is performing a vaginal exam on a pregnant client. She notes a bluish color discoloration of the cervix. The nurse is aware of this is:

    A.   Chloasma sign
    B.   Chadwick's sign
    C.   Goodell's sign
    D.   Braxton's sign

# QUICK FACTS FOR NCLEX QUIZ PAGES 1-20

Directions:
Please do the questions inside the book and enter your answers in your virtual trainer for a score. Once your test is complete, you will not be able to view your exam again. Mark your answers in the book. You will need an 95% to pass the exam.

1. What is the primary physiological dysfunction associated with celiac disease?

    A. Chronic constipation
    B. Inflammation of large intestines
    C. Watery diarrhea
    D. Inability to absorb fat

2. Which of the following is most important when teaching the parents of a child diagnosed with celiac disease?

    A. Tell parents to care for the child's ulcers to avoid infection properly.
    B. Dietary restrictions must be properly managed.
    C. Gluten must be added to maintain a proper healthy balance.
    D. Monitor the physical symptoms associated with a distended abdomen.

3. A nurse is caring for a client who has developed a persistent, nagging cough. Which medication is most likely responsible?

    A. Furosemide
    B. Robitussin
    C. Lisinopril
    D. Klonopin

4. A nurse is administering blood too fast, and the client is experiencing fluid overload. Which symptoms will the client begin to complain of?

    A. Dyspnea, tachycardia, and distended neck veins
    B. Hypotension, oliguria, and urticaria
    C. Shivering, pyrexia, and thirst
    D. Hypothermia, hypotension, and bradycardia

5. A nurse is caring for a client with an abdominal aortic aneurysm. Which of the following will be a part of the treatment plan?

    A. Keep the client on nitroprusside.
    B. A care plan with intravenous fluids for hydration.
    C. A gradual increase in pulsatile flow.
    D. Soft, low fiber diet to prevent constipation and straining.

6. A client is receiving continuous bladder irrigation after a TURP procedure. The nurse is aware the primary goal of the irrigation is which of the following?

    A. To keep the urine light pink.
    B. To reduce bladder spasms.
    C. To reduce the pressure on the prostate.
    D. To reduce the formation of blood clots.

7. A client is experiencing autonomic dysflexia the nurse caring for this client knows which of the following is **most** likely the cause of the medical emergency?

A. Turning the client every 2 hours due to strict bed rest.
B. A colostomy bag that is over full.
C. Administering a vasodilator and increasing blood flow to the brain.
D. Kidney stones from acid salts.

8. A nurse is caring for a client with bell's palsy. Which of the following statements made by the client need follow-up education?

A. The numbness is caused by an interruption of communication in the blood vessels of my face.
B. I can take steroids to reduce some of the swelling I experience.
C. One side of my face may be affected more than the other.
D. A virus may cause the inflammation.

9. After administering a leukotriene modifier, which action should the nurse take?

A. Place the client in a semi-fowlers position.
B. Give the client food to eat.
C. Assess the client's blood pressure.
D. Assess the client for lung sounds and wheezing.

10. A parent has received teaching for childcare for her 4-year-old diagnosed with HIV. Which of the following statements needs follow-up teaching?

A. "I will cover any uneaten food of my child's and place it in the refrigerator."
B. "I will monitor my child's weight."
C. "I will make sure to take out trash weekly."
D. "I should wash my child's eating utensils in the dishwasher with family dishes."

11. Which one of the following HIV medications is a nucleoside reverse transcriptase inhibitor?

A. Famciclovir
B. Norvir
C. Invirase
D. Zidovudine

12. A nurse is caring for a client with an opportunistic infection. What should be included in the treatment plan of a client with Kaposi's sarcoma?

A. A sputum culture to determine the presence of tuberculosis.
B. A screening for lymphomas during the follow-up period.
C. Place the client on contact precautions.
D. Apply a hot moist compress on the skin.

13. A nurse working at a free clinic has been given the assignment of health promotion. When assessing clients in the community, which question should she ask to facilitate HIV health promotion?

A. How many sexual partners do you currently have?
B. Are you able to get access to antiviral medications?
C. When you are sick, are you able to maintain employment?
D. Are you afraid of contracting HIV?

# PHYSIOLOGICAL ASSESSMENT PROGRESS EXAM

Directions:
These are your progress exam questions. Please do the items inside the book and enter your answers in your virtual trainer for a score. Once your test is complete, you will not be able to view your exam again. Mark your answers in the book. You will need an 95% to pass the exam.

1. A 21-year-old male client who has a spinal injury below the level of T6 will most likely have difficulty with:

    A. Mastering his environment.
    B. Identifying with the male role.
    C. Developing meaningful relationships.
    D. Separating himself from his environment.

2. A day after a right hip replacement, a 69-year-old male client remarks to the nurse, "My wife won't like taking care of an old man." These comments by the client regarding himself are an example of Erikson's conflict:

    A. Initiative vs. guilt
    B. Integrity vs. despair
    C. Industry vs. inferiority
    D. Generativity vs. stagnation

3. The nurse should recognize that a genitourinary factor that may contribute to urinary incontinence in the elderly is:

    A. Sensory deprivation
    B. A urinary tract infection
    C. The frequent use of aspirin
    D. Inaccessibility of a bathroom

4. When correcting myths about aging, the nurse should teach that older adults typically have:

    A. A slower reaction time
    B. A negative attitude
    C. Some senile dementia
    D. Confusion at times

5. A 76-year-old female is admitted to the hospital because of complications associated with severe dehydration. The client's son asks the nurse how his mother could have become dehydrated because she is alert and able to care for herself. The nurse's best response would be:

    A. Access to fluid such as water may be limited to meet the daily needs of the older adult.
    B. The body's need for fluid decreases with age due to reduced muscle tissue.
    C. Memory declines with age, and the older adult may forget to ingest adequate amounts of fluids.
    D. The thirst reflex diminishes with age, and therefore the recognition of the need for fluid is decreased.

6. A 78-year-old female client tells the nurse that she read about a vitamin that may be related to aging because of its relationship to the cell wall structure. The client asks if she should be taking it. The nurse is aware the client is referring to:

A. Vitamin E
B. Vitamin C
C. Vitamin A
D. Vitamin K

7. Nursing actions for the older adult include health education and promotion. When dealing with the older adult, the nurse should:

A. Encourage naps and exercise
B. Strengthen the concept of ageism
C. Teach the client about a high-carbohydrate, high fat diet
D. Reinforce the client's strength and promote reminiscing

8. The nurse is aware of the mental process most sensitive to deterioration with aging is which of the following?

A. Creativity
B. Decision-making ability
C. Intelligence
D. Short-term memory

9. A registered nurse is preparing a community health program for senior citizens. The nurse teaches the group that normal physical findings that are expected in older clients include:

A. A gain in skin elasticity and decrease in libido
B. Impaired fat digestion and decreased salivary secretion
C. An increase in body temperature and swallowing difficulties
D. Increased blood pressure and decreased hormone production

10. An 82-year-old male client with osteoporosis is admitted to the hospital with a compression fracture to the spine. The nurse understands that a factor of special concern when caring for the older adult client is which of the following?

A. Inability to remember past facts
B. Irritability
C. Inability to maintain an optimal level of functioning
D. Sudden memory loss due to change in the environment

11. The nurse understands that the first activity of daily living that should be taught to the developmentally disabled child is:

A. Toileting
B. Self-feeding
C. Brushing hair
D. Clapping hands

12. An appropriate toy for a 3-month-old infant would be a:

A. Push-pull toy
B. A plastic mirror
C. Stuffed animal
D. Large plastic ball

13. The nurse is aware that the play of a 5-month old infant is most likely to consist of:

    A. Picking up a rattle or toy and putting it into the mouth
    B. Exploratory searching when a cuddly toy is hidden from view
    C. Simultaneously kicking the legs and waving the hands in the air
    D. Waving and dropping toys placed in the hands

14. A nurse is educating the parents of a 4-year-old child who must be hospitalized for 6 days. During the hospitalization, the nurse is aware the child will probably:

    A. Refuse to cooperate with nurses during the parent's absence.
    B. Demonstrate despair when parents do not visit at least every other day.
    C. Cry when the parents leave and return but cooperate during their absence.
    D. Avoid playing with peers in the playroom.

15. The nurse is caring for a 3-year-old client. Which toy is **most** appropriate?

    A. Rattle
    B. A lunch box filled with large letters
    C. A 7 piece jigsaw puzzle
    D. Blunt scissors and paper

16. When caring for a 4-year-old client, the nurse notes the child stutters. The nurse is aware that stuttering in a 4-year-old child is considered which of the following?

    A. A normal finding for a preschooler.
    B. A sign of a delay in neural development.
    C. The result of an emotional problem.
    D. An indication of serious permanent impairment.

17. The nurse is doing education to parents who are ready to feed their child a variety of solid foods. The infant is on a regular diet. The nurse should encourage the parents to feed the infant, which of the following foods?

    A. Peas, carrots, chicken, and formula
    B. Pears, green beans, ham, and whole milk
    C. Bananas, sweet potatoes, ham, and formula
    D. Peaches, corn, pears, whole milk

18. A nurse is caring for a 2-year-old client diagnosed with lead poisoning. The nurse knows this primarily happens at this age due to:

    A. Lead is easily available.
    B. The vascular system is very fragile.
    C. There is a high level of oral activity in this age group.
    D. Lead pollution has increased.

19. The nurse is aware of the normal development for a 5-year-old is which of the following?

    A. Ritualistic playing
    B. Worries about what his peers will think
    C. Asks for a bottle
    D. Play near others quietly but not with them

20. Which of the following is the **first** step in the nursing health assessment?

    A. Wash the hands.
    B. Greet the client.
    C. Provide privacy.
    D. Obtain consent.

# CLINICAL JUDGEMENT ACTIVITY #7

*Match the abnormal condition with the lesion, organ or body part that is involved with the condition.*

| | |
|---|---|
| 1. Dysplasia | A. Cervical spinal cord lesion |
| 2. Dyspnea | B. Pancreas |
| 3. Quadriplegia | C. Esophagus |
| 4. Diarrhea | D. Lungs |
| 5. Hyperglycemia | E. Urinary bladder |
| 6. Dysphagia | F. Lumbar spinal cord lesion |
| 7. Dysuria | G. Colon |
| 8. Paraplegia | H. Heart |
| 9. Bradycardia | I. brain lesion |
| 10. Aphasia | J. Uterine cervix |
| 11. Hematoma | K. Blood |

Answer Box.   1. J      2. D      3. A      4. G      5. B.      6. C.      7. E      8. F      9. H      10. I      11. K

# DIETS

| Diet | Indication | Food |
|---|---|---|
| | 1.<br><br>Or<br><br>2. | |
| | 1. | Water, juices, see through- broth, |
| | 1. | |
| **Pureed** | 1.<br><br>2. | How should the foods be placed when feeding? |

| | 1. | Any food that can be easily broken down |
|---|---|---|
| **Mechanical Soft** | | |
| | 1. | Can not nave:<br><br><br>Avoid CAP |
| **Protein** _____ | 1. | Avoid:<br><br><br>Why should renal clients avoid protein? |

| | | |
|---|---|---|
| **Restricted** | 1.<br><br><br><br>82 grams or 1 gram<br>heart healthy | |
| | 1. | |
| | 1. | Avoid Purine |
| **High Protein** | 1.<br><br>2. | |
| | 1. | Meal percentages |
| **Celiac** | 1. | Avoid BROW<br><br><br><br>Bread?<br>Spaghetti?<br>Pie?<br>Cookies?<br>Waffles?<br>Pancakes? |

# BASIC CARE & COMFORT

## A. Hygiene

When bathing clients always start with

| 1. Elderly Care | The Skin Is: |
|---|---|
| 2. _____<br><br>_____ Care | _____ and dry feet daily<br>Do not<br>Do not cut:<br>Do not use_____ between the toes<br><br>Check for: |

Who should be delegated to give the client a bath?

## B. Rest

Adequate sleep supports _____ _____.

| Age | NCLEX Notes on Sleep Patterns |
|---|---|
| **Infants 0-1** | _____ to _____ hours each day<br><br>Place infant back to reduce:<br><br>Do not place object (pillows, blankets, toys) in crib |
| **Children 2-8** | _____ to _____ hours each day<br>Naps may be required |
| **Adults** | _____ to _____ hours each day |
| **Elderly** 65+ | Decline in:<br><br>Establish: |

## C. Hydration

To know hydration you have to be able to properly assess dehydration.

_____ is a fluid imbalance.

Signs.

Cardiac Changes:

In dehydration urine levels may drop below the normal:

Common causes of dehydration:

**Treatment:** Rehydration

ReMar's Tip: Oral hydration can be just as effective as IV hydration if started early enough.

NCLEX TIPS:
1. Start with:

2. Do not force _____  _____

3. If oral fluids are not tolerated the next step is:

## D. Bladder & Bowel Elimination

## E. Urine

| | |
|---|---|
| **How much urine is produced each day?** | |
| **Odor?** | |
| **Specific gravity** | 1.016 - 1.022 |
| **pH** | |

**Critical Thinking Question: Why are UTIs more common in women than men?**
**Alteration in normal urine pattern matching**

| | | |
|---|---|---|
| **Anuria** | | A. glucose in the urine |
| **Glycosuria** | | B. involuntary urination at night |
| **Hematuria** | | C. no kidney function |
| **Pyuria** | | D. blood in the urine |
| **Enuresis** | | E. Pus in urine |

NEED TO KNOW NCLEX SKILL: _____

Start with an _____ _____.

Ask patient to void then: throw away.

All _____ must be kept in _____ container.

If one urine sample missed:

Keep _____ on _____.

## Critical Thinking Question

Which of the following is the correct order for the registered nurse to perform an abdominal assessment?

     1. Auscultation, percussion, inspection, and palpation.
     2. Inspection, auscultation, percussion, and palpation.
     3. Inspection, palpation, percussion, and auscultation.
     4. Percussion, inspection, auscultation, palpation.

F. Bowel

| **Handling Normal Stool** | **Which Precaution:** |
|---|---|
| | |

| Factors Affecting Bowel Patterns |
| --- |
| 1. Privacy |
| 2. |
| 3. |
| 4. |
| 5. |

## BASIC CARE & COMFORT

| | |
| --- | --- |
| **Definition of constipation** | |
| **Definition of diarrhea** | |

Bowel Tests to know

| | |
| --- | --- |
| 1. | Screens for: |
| 2. | |

**NCLEX Skills Question:**
The nurse administering an enema to a client knows that the tip of the tubing should be inserted into the rectum while the client is in a sitting position, as on the toilet. True or false?

A. True

B. False

# CLINICAL JUDGMENT ACTIVITY #8

**Draw a line to match the prefix to the correct meaning.**

| | |
|---|---|
| 1. Bio- | A. White |
| 2. Cephalo- | B. Head |
| 3. Erythro- | C. Disease |
| 4. Entero- | D. Life |
| 5. Leuko- | E. Blood |
| 6. Onco- | F. Bone |
| 7. Osteo- | G. Skin |
| 8. Patho- | H. Intestines |
| 9. Hemo- | I. Gland |
| 10. Adeno- | J. Red |
| 11. Dermo- | K. Tumor |

Answer Box:    1. D    2. B.    3. J    4. H    5. A    6. K.    7. F.    8. C    9. E.    10. I.    11. G

# ORTHOPEDICS

**1. Canes**    The cane moves with the _____ _____

then the _____ _____ follows.

**2. Casts**

Use _____ of our hands to handle during first 24 hours.

Do not use _____.

Do not get the cast _____.

What about scratching underneath cast?

Always remember to do _____ _____.

| | |
|---|---|
| **NCLEX Emergency:** | This is an:<br><br>Assess for 6 P's<br><br>1.<br><br>2.<br><br>3.<br><br>4.<br><br>5.<br><br>6.<br><br> Nursing Interventions:<br><br>1. Cast or restricted bandages:<br><br>2. Do not _____   the    _____.<br><br>3.<br><br>*Fasciotomy-surgical decompression is also a possible treatment.<br><br>Why is the urine output so important? |

# ORTHOPEDICS

**3. Crutches-**

Measurements need to be:

Top of crutches should be _____ _____below _____

The handgrips should be:

**Gaits**

Three Point Gait

| 2 Point | Move left crutch with right foot then right crutch with left foot. |
|---|---|
| 3 Point | Move crutches and weaker leg, then strong leg. |
| 4 Point | Move left crutch, then right foot, then right crutch and then follow with the left foot. |
| Swing Through | Move both crutches forward then bear all weight on crutches and swing legs forward at the same time. |

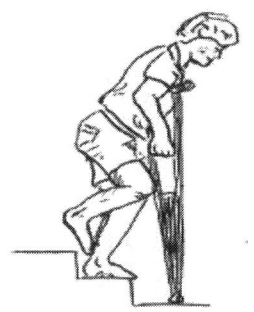

Stair walking with Crutches

| Going up the stairs | |
|---|---|
| Going down the stairs | |

## 4. Walkers-

| Never try to use: |
| Elbows flexed at: |
| Step first with _____ leg then follow with _____ leg. |
| Do not pick: |

| Promoting Circulation | 1. Need _____   _____ |
|---|---|
| Thromboembolic Compression Stockings (TED) | A. Put them on while client is<br><br>_____ _____.<br><br>Time Limit: |
| 2.<br><br>(SCD) | Monitor for: |

**Clients are not allowed to:**

a. Cross their _____.

b. _____ for long:

c. Put _____behind the _____

| Advanced Clinical Topic: | _____is a _____<br><br>_____ _____<br>to limbs, bones, or tissue. |
|---|---|

# ORTHOPEDICS

There are 2 types of _____:

1. _____

Indications:

1. Femoral fractures

2.

3.

The _____ is applied over a _____

_____.

_____ are used to exert a pulling force.

Examples:

Heels should be:
Time Limit:

2. _____

Indications:

1. Fractures of _____

2. Fractures of _____

Metal pins or wires surgically applied.

_____ inserted _____ to_____.

Avoid _____ _____.

Damage _____ in _____.

Notify the healthcare provider if:

1.

2.

## Items Needed for Successful Traction

    A.

    B. Overhead frame

    C. Bars and ropes

    D.


## Client's Activity Level:

## Watch for :

1. _____ bags should hang _____.

2. _____ ropes they should be _____.

3. Watch for _____   _____.

4. _____ due to _____and _____.


## Critical Thinking Questions:

1. A client was hit by a motor vehicle 12 hours ago and is being discharged with a Plaster of Paris cast of the right leg. Which of the following statements need follow-up teaching?

    1. "I will not scratch the skin under my cast."
    2. "I will use the palms of my hands to handle the cast for the next 8 hours."
    3. "I will not get my leg cast wet during basin baths."
    4. "I will notify the healthcare provider if I feel numbness in my leg."

2. A nurse is caring for a client in skeletal traction. Which of the following are expected findings? Select all that apply.

    1. Redness and inflammation at the pin site.
    2. Purulent drainage at the pin site.
    3. Serous drainage at the pin site.
    4. Chest pain due to immobilization.
    5. Loosening of the pin with frequent movement.

3. A nurse is caring for a client with signs of acute compartment syndrome. The client is reporting numbness and tingling in the left lower extremity. Which is the **priority** action of the registered nurse?

    1. Notify the healthcare provider.
    2. Obtain baseline vital signs.
    3. Assess respiratory status.
    4. Assess pedal pulses.

# BASIC CARE & COMFORT HOMEWORK EXAM

> **Directions:**
> These are your progress exam questions. Please do the items inside the book and enter your answers in your virtual trainer for a score. Once your test is complete, you will not be able to view your exam again. Mark your answers in the book. You will need an 95% to pass the exam.

1. A new nurse has just received Mr. Brown to the medical-surgical unit. After the assessment, the nurse notices the client has difficulty speaking, chewing, or swallowing. Which is the best type of diet for Mr. Brown?

   A. Low residue
   B. Clear liquid
   C. Full liquid
   D. Bland
   E. Mechanical soft
   F. High residue

2. The first step in performing any procedure is to:

   A. Obtaining verbal and written consent.
   B. Gathering necessary equipment.
   C. Reviewing the physician's progress report.
   D. Washing the hands.

3. A nurse is feeding an elderly client. The client has a delusion that he is doing karate. He hits the nurse. Which is the **most** appropriate action of the nurse?

   A. Assess the client for delusions.
   B. Call for help.
   C. Administer the prescribed sedative.
   D. Reorient the client to time, place, and situation.

4. A client presents to the emergency department. Which symptom should be reported to the healthcare provider **first**?

   A. Skin that feels hot to the touch.
   B. No bowel movement in the last seven days.
   C. A bluish tint to lips and skin.
   D. Temperature-101. 4, Pulse-88, Respirations-26

5. Mr. Jones, a 60-year-old postoperative client, has his door closed. The registered nurse needs to take a set of routine vital signs. The nurse should do which of the following?

   A. Knock on the door and wait for the client to respond.
   B. Come back in 10 minutes to give the client privacy.
   C. Open the door immediately, as doors should not be closed.
   D. Knock and enter without waiting for a response in case the client is in danger.

6. Which vitamin is most effective in preventing neural tube defects in babies?

    A.   Vitamin D
    B.   Vitamin C
    C.   Niacin
    D.   Folic acid

7. A nurse has just received a newly born infant and knows to prevent heat loss from evaporation by which of the following methods?

    A.   Placing the baby in a warmer after a bath.
    B.   Drying the baby with a soft towel after a bath.
    C.   Monitoring the temperature frequently.
    D.   Placing the crib in the center of the room.

8. A nurse is caring for a newborn baby diagnosed with jaundice. The mother asks the nurse about breastfeeding this baby. The **best** response by the nurse is to tell the mother which of the following?

    A.   The baby should be bottle feed until further testing is done.
    B.   The baby may need to switch to formula while the jaundice is present.
    C.   The baby will need to be fed every 4-6 hours to help rest the stomach.
    D.   The baby should be breastfed every 2-3 hours.

9. At which age will a child not receive the DTap immunization if started on a regular schedule?

    A.   Birth
    B.   2 months
    C.   4 months
    D.   6 months

10. A 4-year-old child refuses to take acetaminophen for a fever. Which nursing strategy would be **most** appropriate?

    A.   Mixing the medication in applesauce so the child is not aware of it.
    B.   Explaining the medication's effects in detail to ensure cooperation.
    C.   Making the child feel ashamed for not cooperating.
    D.   Showing trust in the child's ability to cooperate even with an unpleasant procedure.

11. What is the priority nursing intervention in the immediate phase after a seizure?

    A.   Assess the client's breathing pattern.
    B.   Position the client comfortably.
    C.   Assess the client's vital signs.
    D.   Reorient the client to time, person, and place.

12. A nurse is teaching a client about seizures. Further teaching is needed if the client makes which of the following statements?

    A. Seizures can be caused by low blood sugar.
    B. My mother had seizures because of a large tumor growing in her muscles.
    C. Seizures may be caused by inflammation of the brain, low blood sugar, and head injuries.
    D. Seizures involved my nervous system and require monitoring.

13. A 5-month-old infant is admitted. Upon admission, the nurse assesses her developmental status as appropriate for age. Which of the following is the child **most** likely to be able to do?

    A. Smile in response to mother's face.
    B. Sit with slight support.
    C. Wave bye-bye.
    D. Reach for shiny objects but miss them.

14. The mother of a 2-year-old child asks the nurse how to cope with the child's frequent temper tantrums when he does not get what he wants immediately. What information should the nurse include when responding?

    A. Spanking the child gently.
    B. Explaining to the child why their behavior is wrong.
    C. Ignore the child as long as they are safe.
    D. Giving the child a delicious snack.

15. A school nurse is orienting parents to the daycare unit. A parent asks the nurse "When is an infant's first word typically spoken?" The **best** response by the nurse is:

    A. By ten months.
    B. Between 11 and 13 months.
    C. Between 15-16 months.
    D. After 26 months.

16. A nurse is orienting on a nursery unit. She should be aware newborns show preference for sounds:

    A. That match their native language.
    B. That are always musical in nature.
    C. That is high in pitch.
    D. That matches the normal rhythms of speech.

17. A 27 years old pregnant client is admitted with premature rupture of membranes (PROM). The nurse is aware of the function of the amniotic sac:

    A. It helps the developing fetus maintain an even temperature.
    B. It provides nutrients to the developing fetus.
    C. Filters germs and drugs away from the developing fetus.
    D. The function is not developed until the third trimester.

18. Which of the following is a stage of cognitive development, according to Piaget?

    A. Hypothetical
    B. Preoperational
    C. Fictional
    D. Conceptual
    E. Sensory physical

# BASIC CARE & COMFORT PROGRESS EXAM

1. In providing care for a client being treated for dehydration, which of the following interventions would be **best** delegated to an experienced unlicensed assistive personnel UAP?

    A. Monitor EKG readings.
    B. Obtain vital signs every 30 minutes.
    C. Check for the presence of pedal edema.
    D. Insert an IV line.

2. The nurse on an orthopedic unit receives report on four clients. Who should the nurse assess **first**?

    A. The client who had a total hip replacement 10 hours ago and has had 100 ml of bloody drainage.
    B. The client who had an external fixation device due to a fractured femur and is requesting pain medication.
    C. The client who had an open reduction of a fractured femur 12 hours ago and has developed a rash on the upper arms and abdomen.
    D. The client who had a total hip replacement 4 hours ago with a temperature of 102 degrees.

3. The registered nurse is teaching a client about crutch walking. Which of the following statements if made by the client, indicates a need for further teaching?

    A. "My elbows should be flexed 20 -30 degrees while walking."
    B. "When I climb stairs, I advance my affected leg first, with my crutches."
    C. "I do not apply pressure under my arm when I use my crutches."
    D. "When I am going to sit in a chair I put both crutches in the hand on my unaffected side."

4. A client with end-stage renal disease (ESRD) is scheduled for hemodialysis in one hour. The nurse should notify the primary health care provider that the client has a:

    A. BUN of 65 mg/dl
    B. Creatinine 3.5 mg/dl
    C. Sodium 146 mEq/L
    D. Potassium 6.8 mEq/L

5. A nurse is teaching a new employee class on infant nutrition. The nurse should instruct parents to introduce:

    A. Pureed beef at seven months.
    B. Fruit juices at four months.
    C. Honey-sweet liquids at six months.
    D. Whole milk at ten months.

6. The middle school nurse is talking with the parent of a child with celiac disease. Which of the following statements would require follow-up by the nurse for additional teaching?

    A. We are able to take our child to a soul food restaurant.
    B. My child likes to eat oatmeal and toast for breakfast.
    C. It is fine for my child to continue to eat chicken and rice.
    D. We are able to eat duck and corn for dinner.

7. What should be used to clean the insertion site of an indwelling catheter:

    A. 10 percent bleach solution
    B. Sterile saline
    C. Clean soapy water
    D. Half strength peroxide with water

8. A client is to receive bethanechol chloride for the treatment of chronic acid reflux. The nurse knows an adverse effect of this medication is which of the following:

    A.   Hypotension, diarrhea, urinary frequency.
    B.   Fungal infections, skin rash, swollen glands.
    C.   Liver failure, proteinuria, edema.
    D.   Premature ventricular contractions, angina, hypertension.

9. Which of the following is seen in clients with acid reflux?

    A.   Backflow of gastric contents into the esophagus
    B.   Ascites
    C.   Pyloric stenosis
    D.   Incompetent rectal sphincter

10. How much urine should a client produce each hour?

    A.   15 ml
    B.   30 ml
    C.   60 ml
    D.   80 ml

11. A nurse is assessing the development of a child for a yearly physical exam. The nurse is aware the child should have complete control of her bladder and not experience any incontinence at which of the following age?

    A.   11 months to 1 year-old
    B.   2-3 year-old
    C.   4-6 year-old
    D.   7-8 year-old

12. The nurse is evaluating the tibia of a client who had a cast placed three days ago. The cast over the ankle feels warm to the touch, and the pain is not relieved when the client changes position. The nurse's priority action should be which of the following?

    A.   Obtain an order for new pain medication.
    B.   Administer the prescribed pain medication.
    C.   Document the finding as expected.
    D.   Report the findings to the healthcare provider.

13. The nurse recognizes that a client understands crutch walking with a three-point gait when the client places weight on the:

    A.   Axillary regions
    B.   Palms of the hands
    C.   Feet that are apart
    D.   Palms of the hands and axillary regions

14. When teaching the client with gout about dietary control, the nurse should inform the client to avoid which of the following?

    A.   Eggs
    B.   Shellfish
    C.   Fried poultry
    D.   Cottage cheese

15. A nurse is caring for a client who says she eats a pescatarian diet. Which of the following should not be included in this client's diet?

    A.   Clams
    B.   Fish
    C.   Cheese
    D.   Beef broth

# MEDICATION ADMINISTRATION

Before you give medications check the rights there are many.

1.    Patient              2.    Drug              3.Dose              4. Route

5.    Time              6. Documentation.              7. Allergies & Many more

Verify _____  _____ Before Administration

| PO | PO- Do not crush medications that end in: |
|---|---|
| **PO means by mouth**  **NPO nothing by mouth** | EC  ER  EX  SR  Liquid- |
| **Ear** | Ad**U**lt-  Chil**d**-  Medications should be _____ _____.  How long should the nurse wait before administration drops? |
| **Rectal** | Alternative to _____ or _____ medication administration.  Use a _____ based lubricant  3 types of oral enemas  1.  2.  3.Kayexalate (polystyrene sulfonate)  *Please know the generic name for kayexalate |

| | |
|---|---|
| **Eye** | Avoid the _____. <br><br> Tell client to look up or down? <br><br> Place medication in lower conjunctiva sac <br><br> If eye drops and eye ointments are both prescribed which should be given first? |
| **Gastric Tube** | Check initial placement with _____. <br><br> Assess for _____. <br><br> Delayed gastric emptying. <br>    Greater than 500 hold medication. <br> Medications should be given via _____. <br><br> Do not mix medications give them separately. |
| **Intramuscular (IM)** | Maximum medication in adult muscle: <br><br> Maximum medication in child: <br><br> *Do not aspirate for vaccines. <br><br> Do not give IM injections: <br><br> Inject at _____ degree angle. |
| **Topical** | Applied directly to body surfaces: <br><br> Is Shampoo a topical medication? <br><br> Wash skin daily |

1.

2.

# ANTIBIOTICS

| | Examples | How They Help | How They Harm |
|---|---|---|---|
| 1. | *Vancomycin is not an aminoglycoside but often added because of the similar side effects | | Lab draw to know:<br><br>Peak Draw Time<br>PO:<br><br>IV:<br><br>Trough:<br><br>Antidote:<br><br>Can you administer during pregnancy? |
| 2. | | | Check first for<br><br>_____<br><br>Signs of allergic reactions?<br><br>Antidote:<br><br>Safe during pregnancy? |
| 3. | | *Acne | Children Precaution under 12:<br><br>Food Interactions:<br><br>Safe during pregnancy? |

# ANTIBIOTICS

**Clinical Judgement Practice Questions**

1. A client is scheduled to receive clindamycin at 9:00 am, at which time should the trough level be drawn by the nurse?

    1. 07:30
    2. 08:00
    3. 08:45
    4. 09:00

2. A teenage client has been prescribed a tetracycline for moderate acne. Which of the following statements is the highest priority in the client education about the medication?

    1. "Use sunscreen when you are exposed to direct sunlight."
    2. "Monitor the teeth for color changes."
    3. "Report any signs of hearing loss to the healthcare provider."
    4. "Reduce the amount of fat in your diet to decrease the presence of ketones."

3. A nurse is caring for an elderly client who has pneumonia. The healthcare provider prescribes penicillin PO for 14 days. When the nurse asks the client if she has a penicillin allergy the client states she does not know as she has never taken the medication. Which of the following is the best response by the nurse?

    1. "I will administer this medication and stay with you for monitoring after you take it."
    2. "I will hold the medication and clarify the order with the healthcare provider."
    3. "I will notify the healthcare provider and suggest a different antibiotic."
    4. "I will notify the pharmacist and discuss other alternatives.

# INTRAVENOUS (IV) THERAPY

IV therapy is used to provide:

| Devices used for IV administration |
| --- |
| 1. |
| 2. |

Peripheral catheters cannulas have sizes:

The smaller the number:

IV tubing care

Change all IV tubing within:

IV tubing for blood is changed:

IV tubing for TPN is changed:

# IV COMPLICATIONS

| Complications | Signs | Nursing Interventions |
|---|---|---|
| 1. | | 1. Stop Infusion Immediately<br><br>2.<br><br>3. Elevate extremity.<br><br>4.<br><br>5. Warm compress is more than 30 minutes ago.<br><br>6.<br><br>7.Restart the IV<br>8. Document |
| 2. | | 1. Stop IV infusion.<br>2.<br>3. Elevate extremity<br>4.<br>5. Notify healthcare provider<br>6.<br>7. Document<br>*Some references may say heat is also an acceptable treatment option. |

| NCLEX Emergency | Air _____ |
|---|---|
| **Signs** | 1.<br><br>2.<br><br>3.<br><br>4. |
| **Nursing Interventions** | 1.<br><br>2.<br><br>3. |

## Critical Thinking Question:

1. A client presents to the emergency room after a hit and run accident. The client has sustained massive trauma and is in a hypotensive crisis situation. Which of the following intravenous cannulas will be **most** beneficial for fluid resuscitation?

    1. 22 gauge
    2. 20 gauge
    3. 18 gauge
    4. 14 gauge

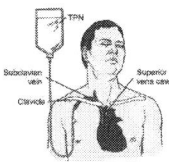 **TOTAL PARENTERAL NUTRITION**

What are the nutrients going through?

Who needs TPN?

Examples

The goal of TPN is to _____ _____.

What labs to monitor?

What electrolyte imbalances can TPN cause?

What is your emergency substitute for TPN?

How do you stop TPN?

**NCLEX Note: How often does the nurse change the tubing?**

# PAIN MANAGEMENT

Pain is _____. It can feel different from client to client.

Pain can be _____ or _____.

| Rating | Technique |
|---|---|
| Adults | |
| Babies/Children | |

**Non-verbal cues of pain**


Pain is experienced differently because of:


Routes for pain medication:


Patient controlled analgesia (PCA) Pump

| NCLEX notes about PCA Pumps. |
|---|


Uses a pump, that delivers medication when the clients wants.

Use for cancer and post-surgical patients.

Critical thinking question:

Should the nurse teach about PCA pump before or after surgery?

| 2 Things to Monitor |
|---|
| 1. |
| 2. |

ReMar Tip: This is a lot of information to learn but you are doing great!

# QUICK FACTS FOR NCLEX 21-40 QUIZ

1. The nurse is caring for a client who has a triglyceride level of 400 and a cholesterol level of 230. Which foods would the nurse encourage in the dietary choices?

    A. Wheat toast and sugar-free jelly.
    B. Grilled salmon seasoned with herbs.
    C. Fried chicken with steamed vegetables
    D. Natural honey from a local farmer's market

2. A nurse is caring for a 22 years old female client who has recently begun dialysis. She asks which types of foods she should avoid into her diet because they are high in potassium. Which of the following should the client be advised to avoid?

    A. cabbage
    B. lean red meat
    C. cooked carrots
    D. avocados

3. A nurse is receiving dietary orders for a newly admitted client. She needs to write for medication to be given "after a meal." Which medical abbreviation should be documented to represent "after a meal?"

    A. AC
    B. PC
    C. TID
    D. HC

4. Dietary recommendations for the client with heart failure include which of the following?

    A. potassium restrictions
    B. protein increase
    C. monitoring fluid intake
    D. addition of salt substitutions

5. The nurse is caring for a client with renal failure. The nurse has an order to consult the dietitian. The dietitian calculates the client's body mass index (BMI) to be 26.9, which of the following categories of weight status would be appropriate to document?

    A. underweight
    B. normal weight
    C. overweight
    D. obese

6. The dietitian is asked to consult with a client who has chronic anemia. This consultation is an example of which of these functions of an inter-professional team?

    A. Standardizing dietary prescriptions.
    B. Individualizing client care.
    C. Utilizing a qualitative descriptive approach.
    D. Ensuring patient adherence to the treatment plan.

7. The nurse is managing a client who is having difficulty following his dietary plan. When preparing to educate the client, the nurse should **first** assess the client's:

    A. medical history.
    B. education level.
    C. learning style.
    D. readiness to learn.

8. During an acute exacerbation of cirrhosis, a client reports ascites. Which of these dietary changes should the nurse expect to be made?

    A.  Increased protein.
    B.  Increased fat.
    C.  Decreased sodium.
    D.  Increased protein.

9. The nurse is administering medication to 4 clients. Which client will need dietary instructions along with their medication?

    A.  The client taking tofranil.
    B.  The client taking senequan.
    C.  The client taking afinitor.
    D.  The client taking phenelzine.

10. A nurse is teaching a client prescribed a monoamine oxidase inhibitor (MAOI). Which foods should be avoided in dietary choices?

    A.  Red wine and pepperoni rolls
    B.  Nacho chips and soda
    C.  Apple pie and strawberry jam
    D.  Orange juice and eggs

11. A client undergoing chemotherapy has frequent episodes of diarrhea. The nurse is aware this is an expected side effect and should encourage which diet?

    A.  A high-protein, high-calorie diet.
    B.  A diet high in fresh fruits and vegetables.
    C.  A diet emphasizing whole and organic foods.
    D.  A bland, low-fiber diet.

12. The nurse is caring for a client with gout. Which of the following dietary selections should the nurse include in the nutritional instructions?

    A.  liver
    B.  sardines
    C.  tuna
    D.  macaroni and cheese
    E.  deer meat

13. A nurse is doing a home health visit for a client with osteoporosis. The nurse should provide which dietary instruction?

    A.  Include dairy products in your planned meals.
    B.  Avoid seeds and nuts.
    C.  Fruits and vegetables will decrease the bone pain.
    D.  Avoid fish foods and shrimp.

14. The student nurse is teaching the family of a client diagnosed with liver failure. She should instruct them to limit which foods in the client's diet?

    A.  Cookies and cakes
    B.  Meats and beans
    C.  Potatoes and pasta
    D.  Butters and dairy

15. The **most** appropriate diet for the client with Meniere's disease is:

    A.  Restricted in sodium
    B.  Restricted in animal fat
    C.  Restricted in protein
    D.  Restricted in gluten

# SUBSTANCE ABUSE

| Substance Abuse | Continued use of a substance |
|---|---|

Substance abuse can be _____ An _____ is considered a _____

_____.

**Substances that are abused are:**

**Clients are at risk for:** Suicide and Overdose

| A. Alcoholism- |
|---|
| **Signs:** |
| **Most alcoholics are in:** |
| **Withdrawal symptoms:** |
| 🛑 **Medical Emergency** |

**Delirium tremors:**

    1. Physical shaking
    2.
    3.
    4.
    5.

2 Other Symptoms to Know

| 1. | |
|---|---|
| 2. | |

🛑 **Medical Emergency**

**Delirium tremors Treatment:**

**Medicate with anti-anxiety medication such as:**

      1.

      2.

      or

      **Alcohol deterrent medications such as:**

      1.

| Teaching point: | Clients must avoid: |
|---|---|

**NCLEX Pro Tip:**

**Medications that contain alcohol:**

**Other therapy options:** Non-judgmental attitude, Support groups Alcoholics anonymous

      There is no _____.

      Clients can be placed in a _____ _____.

# SUBSTANCE ABUSE

| B. Opioid Addiction |
|---|
| Examples: |
| Room Assignment: |
| Withdrawal Symptoms: |

_____: is a legal narcotic that can be used as a substitute.

# IV FLUIDS

There are _____ _____of intravenous fluids.

**NCLEX Pro Tip**: All 3 are used to treat some form of _____.

| IV Fluids | Examples |
|---|---|
| 1. _____<br><br>Lower:<br>1. Osmotic Pressure<br><br><br>2. Concentration of<br><br><br><br>Pulls fluid: | What type of dehydration does this treat?<br><br>Also used for:<br><br>Avoid:<br><br>Clients with decreased renal function<br>Clients with:<br>Clients with: |
| 2. _____<br><br>Same:<br>1.<br><br><br>2.<br><br><br>Does not draw or push fluid into the cell. | What type of dehydration does this treat?<br>Intravascular dehydration<br>Also used for:<br><br><br>Avoid clients with:<br><br>1. Decreased renal function<br>2. Cardiac disease |
| 3. _____<br>Higher:<br>1.<br>2.<br> Does not draw or push fluid into the cell.<br>*Avoid:*<br>*Clients with compromised renal functions*<br>*Clients with congestive heart failure*<br>*Clients with diabetic ketoacidosis* | 5%NS<br>D5%NS<br>D5LR<br>10% Dextrose in Water D10W<br><br>What type of dehydration does this treat?<br>Intravascular dehydration w/ cellular over hydration<br>Used for: |

**General Nursing Intervention Tips:**

# CLINICAL MATH

**Florence Nightingale:**

**Mother of modern nursing**

**NCLEX Units of Measurements**

| |
|---|
| **There will be no complex math during this study session.** |
| **This math will be based off the Quick Facts for NCLEX book.** |

**A. Working with Numbers:**

_____ describe _____ _____.

**Example:** height, weight, blood pressure.

These numbers can be _____ or _____.

---

**Calculating Fluid Balance**

Formula:

Can a client's fluid balance be negative?

What does this mean?

A client's intake is 800 mL.

The same client's output is 2000 mL.

What is the net fluid balance of this client?

---

**Critically think:**
Which types of clients need negative fluid balances?

      1.

      2.

      3.

Watch for these clients with negative fluid balances (not helpful)

4. Dementia, Alzheimer's

# CLINICAL MATH

5.

**B. Multiplication:**

Let's Work!

Multiplying by _____.

| 79 x 0 | |
|---|---|
| 6 x 0 | |
| 144 x 0 | |

Multiplying by _____.

| 12.5 x 1 | |
|---|---|
| 4 x 1 | |
| 62 x 1 | |

Multiplying by _____.

| 12 x 10 | |
|---|---|
| 83 x 10 | |
| 95 x 10 | |

Multiplying by one _____.

| 10 x 100 | |
|---|---|
| 35 x 100 | |

Metric system uses multiples of _____.

**C. Division:**

In medical math division is represented by a _____.

$12 \div 3 = 4$ or $\dfrac{12}{3} = 4$

$10 \div 2 = 5$ or $\dfrac{10}{2} = 5$

$24 \div 8 = 3$ or $\dfrac{24}{8} = 3$

**Real Life Practice:**

1. A client is prescribed 750 mg of lansoprazole per day. The medication comes in 250 mg tablets. How many tablets will be administered per day?

Remember _____ just means a part of a _____.

| ¼ |
|---|
| 0.50 |
| 1:8 |
| 35% |

These are all _____.

**Reduce these fractions to the lowest terms:**

| | |
|---|---|
| 1.    $\dfrac{10}{20}$ | |
| 2.    $\dfrac{5}{15}$ | |
| 3.    $\dfrac{4}{32}$ | |

## D. Conversions: _____System

Metric system is easy because it uses _____math.

| | |
|---|---|
| **mili**   1/1000   or 0.001 | |
| **centi**   1/100   or 0.01 | |
| **deci**   1/10    or 0.1 | |

| | |
|---|---|
| **Confusion Alert:** | Another name for the metric system |

## E. System:

| Weight | Liquids |
|---|---|
| | Cup |
| | Fluid oz. (fl oz.) |
| | Tablespoon (Tbsp) |
| | Teaspoon (Tsp. |
| | Drop (gtt) |

What about the apothecary system? Examples are listed here these will not be found on the NCLEX but you should be familiar with the name for historical reference.

| | | | |
|---|---|---|---|
| **Drams.** | **Scrumple.** | **Grains.** | **Minim.** |

Most conversion problems require you to remember _____ _____.

| Metric Unit | Household Unit | | |
|---|---|---|---|
| 1 mL | | | |
| 5 mL | | | |
| 15 mL | | | |
| 30 mL | | | |
| 237 or 240 mL | | | |
| 1 kg | | | |

Record ice chips _____

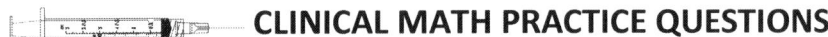 

CRITICALLY THINK

1. If a client took 6 oz. of ice chips, how many mLs of fluid should the nurse record?

2. A client is prescribed simethicone 30 mL PO BID. The medication comes in 50mg/500 mL. How many teaspoons are in each dose?

3. Which client is most appropriate to take a medication in the form of a liquid? Select all that apply.

      1-A. A 26-years-old with a compromised IV site.
      2-B. A 9-month-old with depressed fontanelles.
      3-C. A 9-years-old with celiac disease.
      4-D. A 43-years-old client newly diagnosed with stroke.
      5-F. A 63-years-old client on strict bed rest.

## Dosage Calculations

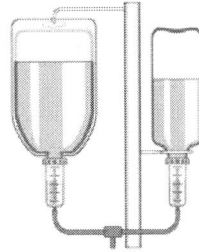

2. A nurse is instructed to administer heparin with a weight-based protocol. The client weighs 220 lbs. She must give 80 units/kg bolus and then start an infusion at 18 units/kg/hr. The heparin comes in 25,000 units in 500 mL of 0.9 NS.

A. What is the client's weight in kilograms?

B. Calculate the bolus dose?

3. Calculate the flow rate?

Flow rate can also be called _____ _____.

Infusions can be _____ or _____.

# CLINICAL MATH

| Simple Formula for Calculating Flow Rate |
|:---:|

Flow rate =

Example: A client is to receive 500 mL of D5 0.45% NaCL over 24 hours. Calculate the IV flow rate.

So for our example using the formula we would write.

Step 1
Flow rate =

| Simple Formula for Calculating Flow Rate |
|:---:|

Flow rate = Total <u>Volume</u>
                        Time

3. A client is ordered 1200 mL D5W IV. The IV solution is to infuse over 10 hours by an infusion pump. Calculate the flow rate in milliliters per hour.

| Conversion Factor: Minutes to Hours |
|:---:|

Formula

4. A nurse is scheduled to administer ketamine 800 mL IV. The IV solution is to infuse over 240 minutes. Calculate the flow rate in milliliters per hour.

| Simple formula for calculating the drip rate |
|:---:|

Drip rate (gtt/min)=

5. A nurse is working in a portable hospital tent. She is working with a manual IV infusion system. Her client must receive 0.9 NS 1000 mL IV over 12 hours. The drop factor is 20 gtt/mL. Calculate the drip rate.

| Simple Formula to Calculate Units per Hour |
|:---:|

6. A client's heparin drip is infusing at 11 mL/hr. on an infusion pump. The premixed solution is 25,000 units of heparin in 250 mL D5W. What hourly dose of heparin is the client receiving?

Step 1.
Find out how many units are in 1 ml.

Heparin Units= units in mL
Volume (mL)

Step 2.

# PHARMACOLOGICAL & PARENTERAL THERAPIES HOMEWORK EXAM

1. A nurse is scheduled to administer an antibiotic to a client who reports being allergic to antibiotics. Which is the **initial** action of the nurse?

    A. Ask the client if they have ever taken the prescribed medication.
    B. Question the client about allergies to other medications.
    C. Request an order for diphenhydramine.
    D. Request to give a smaller dose of the medication.

2. The nurse is caring for a newly admitted client who drinks grapefruit juice every morning. The nurse will be concerned about which class of medication due to a possible interaction?

    A. Acetaminophen
    B. Penicillin
    C. Aminoglycosides
    D. Calcium channel blockers

3. A client taking oral contraceptives is concerned her other prescribed medications may decrease the effects of birth control. She does not want to become pregnant. Which question should the nurse ask to evaluate the possible risk of pregnancy?

    A. "Do you take vitamin C daily?"
    B. "Do you take seizure medication?"
    C. "Do you drink grapefruit juice?"
    D. "Do you take your oral contraceptives with milk?"

4. A nurse working on a pediatric unit is preparing to administer penicillin G intramuscularly to a 4-years-old child. The child's parents ask why the drug cannot be given by mouth. Which is the correct response by the nurse?

    A. "This drug causes severe gastric upset if given orally."
    B. "This drug has a narrow therapeutic range, and the dose must be tightly controlled."
    C. "This drug is absorbed much too quickly in an oral form."
    D. "Enzymes in the stomach would inactivate this drug."

5. A client has been receiving penicillin for chlamydia for several days and begins to complain of generalized hives. The client also states his skin is itching. Which is the **most** appropriate action by the nurse?

    A. Administer the next dose and continue to evaluate the client's symptoms.
    B. Ask the prescriber if an antihistamine can be given to relieve the itching.
    C. Hold the next dose and obtain blood and urine cultures.
    D. Hold the next dose and notify the healthcare provider of the symptoms.

6. A nurse is preparing to administer medications to a group of clients. Which client is **most** at risk for an adverse reaction?

    A. A 19-years-old with kidney disease.
    B. A 65-years-old with dementia.
    C. An 83-years-old with cystitis.
    D. A 50-year-old man with an upper respiratory tract infection.

7. A licensed practical nurse is ordered to give morphine 5 mg PO every 12 hours PRN for pain. Which action is not part of the six rights of drug administration?

    A. Checking the medication administration record to see when the last dose was administered.
    B. Assessing the client's pain level 15 to 30 minutes after giving the medication.
    C. Consulting a drug manual to determine whether the amount the prescriber ordered is appropriate.
    D. Documenting the reason the medication was given in the client's electronic medical record.

8. A client with terminal cancer reports pain; the client rates the pain as a seven on a scale from 0 to 10. The healthcare prescriber has ordered acetaminophen 650 mg PO every 8 hours PRN pain. Which action should the nurse take?

    A. Ask the client what medications have helped with pain in the past.
    B. Contact the healthcare provider to request a different pain medication.
    C. Give the pain medication and reposition the client to promote comfort.
    D. Request an order to administer the medication every 6 hours.

9. A 22-years-old client is using a metered-dose inhaler containing albuterol for asthma. The medication label instructs the client to administer "2 puffs every 8 hours as needed." The client reports feeling dizzy sometimes when taking the medication, and she doesn't think that the medication is always effective. Which action is outside the nurse's scope of practice?

    A. Asking the client to demonstrate the use of the inhaler.
    B. Assessing the client's exposure to tobacco smoke.
    C. Auscultating lung sounds and obtaining vital signs.
    D. Suggesting that the client use one puff to reduce side effects.

10. A nurse is providing care to a client who is receiving heparin via an intravenous infusion. He reports chest pain and chills. His temperature is elevated, as is his heart rate. He has developed a red skin rash. The client's signs and symptoms are consistent with which of the following?

    A. DKA
    B. HIT
    C. DVT
    D. pulmonary embolism

11. The healthcare provider has ordered a medication that is to be administered once per day in the morning. It should be noted as which of the following?

    A. a.c.
    B. q.a.m
    C. q.d.
    D. o.a.m.

12. A client treated in the cardiac unit has received education on the use of nitroglycerin. The licensed vocational nurse determines follow-up teaching is effective if the client makes which of the following statements?

    A. "If I experience chest pain, I should contact my doctor right away."
    B. "I can take another nitroglycerin in 20 minutes if the pain does not go away."
    C. "If I have chest pain, I should stop my activity and take a nitroglycerin tablet."
    D. "If I have chest pain, I should rest for 30 minutes and then take a nitroglycerin tablet."

13. When planning emergent care for a client with a suspected myocardial infarction, which of the following should the nurse anticipate administrating?

    A. Oxygen, furosemide, nitroglycerin, and meperidine.
    B. Oxygen, nitroglycerin, aspirin, and morphine.
    C. Aspirin, nitroprusside, dopamine, and oxygen.
    D. Nitroglycerin, lorazepam, oxygen, and warfarin

14. The healthcare provider prescribes clonidine 0.4 mg PO twice daily for three days. The pharmacy has clonidine 0.1 mg tablets available.
Calculate the daily dose. _____

15. A client is prescribed ampicillin 250 mg PO four times a day for 10 days. The pharmacy has 125 mg per 5 mL on hand.

Calculate the complete dose given in the 10 days in milliliters. _____

# PHARMACOLOGICAL & PARENTERAL THERAPIES PROGRESS EXAM

1. A client with congestive heart failure is being treated with diuretic therapy. Which of the following assessments **best** indicate to the nurse that the client's condition is improving?

    A.   The client has an increase in urinary output.
    B.   The client's blood pressure has decreased.
    C.   The client is requesting fluids as the medication is effective.
    D.   The client has fewer crackles during auscultation.

2. The nurse is treating a client with a standing PRN order for hydromorphone every four hours for surgical pain. Which of the following assessments would indicate the nurse should discontinue the medication?

    A.   The client complains of a burning sensation during IV administration.
    B.   The client's respiratory rate is 13 breaths per minute.
    C.   The client's blood pressure is 80/68.
    D.   The client reports a decreased appetite.

3. A client is discharged home with an enteral feeding tube. Which action should the home health nurse perform to determine the patency of the client's enteral tube?

    A.   Instill air into the tube to check for placement and patency before each feeding.
    B.   Auscultate the client's abdomen for bowel sounds before each feeding.
    C.   Arrange for the client to have an x-ray performed periodically.
    D.   Test aspirated tube contents for pH level before each feeding.

4. A client who is receiving nutrition via a percutaneous endoscopic gastrostomy tube exhibits nausea and vomiting. The client states his heart feels like it is racing. Which of the following should the nurse expect?

    A.   Refeeding syndrome
    B.   Abdominal distention
    C.   Hypokalemia
    D.   Aspiration pneumonia

5. A nurse is caring for a client who has experienced an allergic reaction to a unit of packed red blood cells. After turning off the intravenous infusion, which action should the nurse take?

    A.   Check the client's vital signs.
    B.   Notify the healthcare provider.
    C.   Maintain an intravenous (IV) infusion of 0.9% sodium chloride.
    D.   Collect blood and urine specimens

6. A nurse is preparing to administer fresh frozen plasma to a client after assessing the vital signs. Which action should she include in her care?

    A.   Obtain Y tubing set and prime with normal saline.
    B.   Plan to assess vital signs again and remain with the client 10 minutes after the infusion starts.
    C.   Set infusion pump to deliver a unit in 1 hour.
    D.   Slow infusion immediately if allergic reactions occur.

7. A nurse is teaching the parents of a child with severe allergies about using the epinephrine pen injection. Which of the following is the correct statement?

    A. The injection should be given in the upper arm.
    B. The injection should be given in the mid-thigh area.
    C. The injection should be given subcutaneously in the inner arm.
    D. The medication is given as an aerosol solution.

8. A nurse is caring for a client admitted to the emergency department. The client was bitten by a stray dog while riding a motorcycle. The client crashed into a tree and has multiple arm fractures and a suspected head injury. Which medication should the nurse expect to administer?

    A. Furosemide
    B. Morphine
    C. Estazolam
    D. Tetanus toxoid

9. A nurse is caring for a client who is experiencing vomiting due to digoxin toxicity. Which medication should the nurse prepare to administer?

    A. Lidocaine
    B. Lisinopril
    C. Atropine
    D. Amlodipine

10. A nurse is planning education for a client who has recently been diagnosed with myasthenia gravis. While discussing the pharmacological therapies, which is the **most** important point to include in the client education?

    A. Take the medication with a full glass of water.
    B. Eat meals during the peak of the medication time.
    C. Take medication early in the day before 9:00.
    D. Avoid citrus fruits when taking medication.

# EASY NCLEX LABS

| Labs | Purpose | Values |
|------|---------|--------|
| **Hemoglobin Hgb** | Transport oxygen to tissue and Co2 back to lungs. RBC's are made up of hemoglobin. If this is Low think Iron deficiency anemia | -male    14-16.5 g/dl<br>-female   12-15 g/dl |
| **Red blood cells RBC** | These carry oxygen from the lungs to the tissues around your body. | -male    4.5-6.2 %<br>-female   4-5.5 % |
| **Hematocrit** | The hematocrit is the ratio of the volume of packed red blood cells to the total blood volume. If it's Low than that indicates a decrease in O2 capacity. | -male    41-51%<br>-female   36-46% |
| **White Blood Cells**<br><br>**WBC** | This is the body's defense against infectious organisms and foreign substances. Chemotherapy would make this laboratory value decreased. | 5,000-10,000 /uL or mm3 |
| **K** | Potassium is a mineral & electrolyte<br>Carries an electrical charge important for many cardiac functions. | 3.5-5.1 mEq/L |
| **Na** | Sodium maintains fluid levels, muscle and nerve functions. | 135-145 mEq/L |
| **Ca** | Calcium is a mineral and electrolyte that is important in bone and teeth development | 8.6-10 mEq/L |
| **Mg** | Magnesium is important for nerves and muscles. It helps neutralize acid in the stomach<br>An example of a medication that contains magnesium is<br>Milk of magnesia (laxative) | 1.6-2.6 mEq/L |
| **Cl** | Chloride keeps the fluid balance in/out of cells in check. We get most of chloride from the sodium chloride we eat. It is digested in the intestines. | 95-105 mEq/L |
| **CO2** | Carbon dioxide is a waste product of the respiratory system but also is necessary for our body to function properly. | 22-32 mEq/L |

| | | |
|---|---|---|
| **BUN** <br> **Blood urea nitrogen** <br> **Liver/kidney test** | The test measures the level of urea in the blood. Urea is a waste product that comes from protein. It's what is left over. Urea is made in the liver but then it is the kidneys' responsibility to get rid of it through the urine. | 8-25 mg/dL (microgram/deciliter) |
| **Creatinine** | This is a test of kidney function. The creatinine clearance rate helps to estimate the glomerular filtration rate (GFR) | 0.6-1.3 mg/dL <br> High creatinine signals renal failure |
| **Liver Enzymes** | 1. aspartate aminotransferase (AST or SGOT) enzyme that is released when the liver or muscle cells are injured. <br><br> 2. alanine aminotransferase (ALT) (Sgpt) like AST this is an enzyme that is found in the liver that is normally low but when liver damage has occurred this value will be elevated. | 1. 10 to 40 IU/L. <br> 2. 5-35 U/L <br><br> These values elevate with hepatitis or jaundice. |
| **Glucose** | Serum glucose is the amount of sugar in the blood. Most of our sugar comes from carbohydrates. | 70-110 mg/dL |
| **PTT** <br> **Partial** <br> **Thromboplastin** <br> **Time** | A blood test that helps doctors assess the body's ability to form a blood clot. The test measures how many seconds it takes for a clot to form. | Clotting should occur in 60-70 seconds <br><br> If the client is taking an anticoagulant it will be 1.5 x 2.5 times longer 120 to 140 seconds. |
| **aPTT** <br> **Activated** <br> **partial** <br> **thromboplastin** <br> **time** | A blood test that is also used to measure the time it takes for a clot to form however an activator is added to the blood that speeds up the clotting time. This test is used mostly to monitor a client's response to heparin. | 30 to 40 seconds <br><br> If the client is taking an anticoagulant it will be 1.5 x 2.5 times longer 60 to 80 seconds. |
| **INR** <br> **international** <br> **normalized ratio** | This is a blood test to determine the clotting time when a client is on an anticoagulant usually vitamin K antagonists such as warfarin. | 1-2 <br><br> 2.0 to 3.0 is standard for clients taking warfarin. |
| **Urine specific gravity** | This is done to test kidney function. This test looks at all of the particles in the urine. | 1.016-1.022 <br><br> Urine sample collection 1 to 2 oz. first thing in the am. |
| **Platelets** | Smallest of the 3 major types of blood cells. Which are red, white, and platelets. <br><br> The function is to prevent bleeding. | 150,000-400,000 µL microliter |

# CLINICAL JUDGEMENT ACTIVITY #9

Write the correct letter of the correct laboratory value to match the term.

|  |  |
|---|---|
| 1. Sodium_____ | A. 14-16.5 |
| 2. Hemoglobin (Male)_____ | B. 0.6-1.35 |
| 3. White blood cells_____ | C. 150,000-400,000 |
| 4. Potassium_____ | D. 8.6-10 |
| 5. Calcium_____ | E. 5,000-10,000 |
| 6. Magnesium_____ | F. 135-145 |
| 7. Chloride_____ | G. 1.016-1.022 |
| 8. BUN_____ | H. 70-110 |
| 9. Glucose_____ | I. 12-15 |
| 10. Phosphorus_____ | J. 7.35-7.45 |
| 11. Platelets_____ | K. 1.6-2.6 |
| 12. Hemoglobin (female)_____ | L. 22-26 |
| 13. Creatinine_____ | M. 8-25 |
| 14. Urine Specific Gravity_____ | N. 95-105 |
| 15. pH_____ | O. 2.5-4.5 |
| 16. $HCO_3$_____ | P. 3.5-5.1 |

Answer box

1. F    2. A    3. E    4. P    5. D    6. K    7. N    8. M    9. H

10. O    11. C    12. I    13. B    14. G    15. J    16. L

# EASY ELECTROLYTES

| Electrolyte | Hyper Signs | Hypo Signs |
|---|---|---|
| 1. Potassium<br><br>Never give<br><br>_____ | Treatment:<br><br>1.<br>2.<br>3.<br><br>*Again please note the generic name is sodium polystyrene. | Treatment:<br><br><br>High potassium foods: |
| 2. | What glands help absorb calcium?<br><br>Treatment: | 3 T's<br><br>Treatment: |

| | | |
|---|---|---|
| 3. | Hypotension<br>Drowsiness<br>Decreased respirations<br>Bradycardia<br><br>Treatment: | Convulsions<br>Seizures<br>Tachycardia<br>High blood pressure<br><br>Treatment: |
| 4. | | |
| 5.<br><br>Think | soDium<br><br><br>Treatment: | sOdium<br><br><br>Treatment: |

# DIABETES INSIPIDUS VS. SYNDROME OF INAPPROPRIATE ANTIDIURETIC HORMONE SECRETION

Both are a problem with:

Diabetes Insipidus

1. Diabetes Insipidus is too little _____.

Signs of diabetes insipidus are:

Will the blood pressure high or low?
Will the Heart rate be increased or decreased?

Treatment:

Syndrome of Inappropriate ADH

2. _____-is too much _____.

Signs of SIADH are:  Oliguria

Sodium level up or down?

Treatment:

# POSITIONS

| 1. Fowler's | 4 types of Fowler's |
| --- | --- |
| | Low-_____ degrees |
| | Semi- _____degrees |
| | Standard-_____ degrees |
| | High-_____degrees |
| | Low fowler's: |
| | Semi: |
| | Standard: |
| | High: |
| 2. | |
| | This position is for: |
| 3. | |
| | What is this client at risk for due to being in this position for a long time? |

| | |
|---|---|
| 4. | Do not put clients who have:<br><br>1.<br><br>2.<br><br>3.<br><br>. |
| 5. | |
| 6. | |
| 7. | |

# DISASTER MANAGEMENT

| _____ Disasters | _____ Disasters |
|---|---|
| Internal happen _____ the<br><br>_____ environment.<br><br>Examples<br><br><br><br><br>Client priority is based on: | _____ disasters happen<br><br>_____ of the facility but will cause a<br><br>_____  _____ of<br><br>people to need medical care.<br><br>Examples<br><br>Client priority use:<br><br>A-<br><br>B-<br><br>C- |

**RN Task what does it mean to triage:**_____

Disaster Management.   _____  _____ _Coded System of_ _____

|  |  |
|---|---|
|  |  |
|  | Bodily injuries but the client is stable. |
|  |  |
|  |  |

Discharge Rules

| Use the other ABCs | Who goes home or get relocated to make room for new clients<br>1.<br>2.<br>3. |
|---|---|

# CLINICAL JUDGEMENT ACTIVITY #10

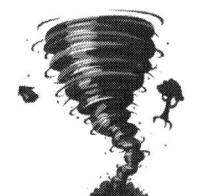

***Choose the correct answer to the disaster related question.***

1. A nurse is caring for a client with a survivable but life threating injury. Using the color coded system she should classify the client as which of the following?

    1. Black
    2. Yellow
    3. Green
    4. Red

2. A nurse is caring for a client with an acute psychological disturbance. Using the color coded system she should classify the client as which of the following?

    1. Red
    2. Yellow
    3. Green
    4. Black

3. The nurse is caring for a client with exposure to the biological agent anthrax. Exposure by which form is most severe:

    1. ingestion
    2. skin contact
    3. inhalation
    4. transcutaneous

4. A nurse is caring for a client who was involved in a bioterrorist attack. The laboratory results determine the agent used inhibits acetylcholinesterase. The nurse should determine this is a:

    1. vesicant
    2. nerve agent
    3. blood agent
    4. sulfur agent

---

Answer box
1. Red is used for clients who require immediate intervention and life threatening injuries.
2. Based on the color coded system the client would be considered green. Minor bodily injury or walking but wounded.
3. Inhalation of the biological agent anthrax is the most severe.
4. An agent that inhibits acetylcholinesterase will disturb actions on the nervous system.

# QUICK FACTS FOR NCLEX PAGES 40-66 QUIZ

1. A mother diagnosed with shingles is concerned that her 2-year-old child is at risk for contracting the virus. The mother states the child has never had varicella-zoster. Which statement should the nurse make?

    A. "No, the child is not at risk."
    B. "Yes, the child is at risk."
    C. "If the child has been exposed to the herpes virus they are more at risk."
    D. "Yes if the child is exposed to open lesions, they are at risk."

2. A mother who practices the Roman Catholic faith is preparing her child for death. The child is expected to live only 8 more hours. Which action should the nurse take?

    A. Not suggest any blood or blood products.
    B. Prepare the client for infant baptism.
    C. Only allow other Roman Catholics to touch the dead body.
    D. Call the Rabbi to give the last sacrament before death.

3. Which statement is true concerning lithium?

    A. Give this medication with food.
    B. The therapeutic drug range is 2.5-3.0 mEq/L.
    C. The medication will work within 72 hours.
    D. This medication can be stopped abruptly.

4. The nurse should monitor the client receiving valproic acid for which adverse effect?

    A. Hypertension
    B. Psychosis
    C. Abdominal cramping
    D. Nose bleeds

5. A nurse is preparing to administer methylergonovine 0.2 mg to a client who is experiencing postpartum bleeding. Which of the following actions should the nurse implement **first**?

    A. Check the client's blood pressure.
    B. Check the client's temperature.
    C. Check the fetal heart rate.
    D. Obtain the client's hemoglobin level.

6. Polystyrene sulfonate is used in renal failure to:

    A. Correct acidosis.
    B. Reduce poison from lead ingestion.
    C. Prevent constipation from a bowel obstruction.
    D. Reduce potassium from the bowels.

7. The nurse is preparing to administer spironolactone to a client. Which diagnosis would refute the order to administer this medication?

    A. Hypokalemia
    B. Heart disease
    C. Benign prostate hypertrophy
    D. Diabetes mellitus

8. A 16-years-old client is diagnosed with a seizure disorder which is being treated with medication. Which of the following medications would the nurse question if ordered for the client?

    A. Phenobarbitol, 150 mg before bed
    B. Amitriptyline, 10 mg four times a day
    C. Valproic acid, 150 mg twice daily
    D. Phenytoin (Dilantin), 100 mg three times a day

9. A client is prescribed cetirizine PO by the healthcare provider. The nurse administering the medication should perform which of the following actions?

    A. Do not give this medication with food.
    B. Do not give this medication if the client has a temperature over 100.0 C.
    C. Do not give this medication if the client is pregnant.
    D. Do not give this medication if the client is allergic to sulfa drugs.

10. When caring for a client with a tracheostomy, which device must always be present at the bedside in case the tracheostomy tube becomes dislodged?

    A. Air-inlet valve
    B. Pilot cuff
    C. Fenestration
    D. Obturator

11. Which of the following clients is **most** appropriate for total parenteral nutrition?

    A. A client with multiple mouth ulcers from throat cancer.
    B. The client with a short bowel obstruction.
    C. The client who has failed several swallowing tests.
    D. The client with severe nausea and vomiting on a clear liquid diet

# HERBAL MEDICATIONS

| Herbal | Action | Client Teaching |
|---|---|---|
| **1. St. John's Wort**<br><br>**Psychiatric Medication** | | Do not give with SSRIs |
| **2.** | | Do not use with anticoagulants |
| **3.** | | |
| **4.** | Seasonal Flu | |
| **5.** | | |
| **6.** | Alleviate menopausal symptoms | |
| 7. | | Hepatotoxic |
| 8. | Benign prostate hypertrophy (BPH) | *erectile dysfunction |

## General Client Teaching:

No _____ needed.

May interact with other medicines

The quality, purity, and _____ may vary.

If surgery is planned stop taking _____ _____ before.

# CLINICAL JUDGEMENT ACTIVITY #11

**Based on the client's statement circle which herbal medication is being administered.**

Client 1.) "Nurse I have noticed an decrease in my depression."

        A. Saw palmetto    B. St. John's Wort    C. Aloe

Client 2.) "Nurse my cholesterol is doing just fine."

        A. Garlic    B. Black cohosh    C. Echinacea

Client 3.) "Nurse my memory has improved since starting this new medication."

        A. Gingko biloba    B. Angelica    C. Bilberry

Client 4.) "Nurse after doing that healthy living challenge my prostate is doing well"

        A. Cranberry    B. Saw palmetto    C. Cat's claw

Client 5.) "Hold the promethazine, I am no longer nauseated after taking this?"

        A. Kava kava    B. Evening primrose    C. Ginger

Client 6.) "Nurse my hot flashes have improved, you can turn off the fan."

        A. Black cohosh    B. Aloe    C. Vitamin C

| Answer box. | 1. B | 2. A | 3. A | 4. B | 5. G. | · 6. A |
|---|---|---|---|---|---|---|

---

**Note to You As a ReMar Nurse!**

You are doing great! Yes this is a lot! But guess what?
Good things come after hard work! Everything you want in life you can have but you have to put in work. Take a deep breath and let's get back to it!

# BLOOD GAS INTERPRETATION BY NUMBERS

| pH | HCO3 |
|---|---|
| elow 7.35=<br><br>bove 7.45 = | |

### THINK R.O.M.E.!     Respiratory Opposite Metabolic Equal

A.) How would you interpret this blood gas? pH 7.53 PaCO2 33  HCO3 33  PaO2 72

pH ⬆ 7.53    HCO3 33    = _____  _____

B.) How                   would you interpret this blood gas?  pH 7.10 PaCO2 24 HCO3 45 BE 3

pH 7.10 _____ HCO3 45 _____ = _____  _____

C.) How would you interpret this blood gas? pH 7.32 PaCO2 35 HCO317 PaO2 89

pH 7.32 _____HCO3  17_____= _____  _____


# BLOOD GAS INTERPRETATION BY DIAGNOSIS

## 1st question: Is this a breathing problem?

| | |
|---|---|
| | M |
| espiratory Alkalosis=<br><br>espiratory Acidosis= | Metabolic Alkalosis-<br><br>Metabolic Acidosis= |

## Critically Think:

1) Which blood gas value would you expect to see in a client with a pulmonary embolus
2)  Which blood gas value would you expect to see in a client who has diabetes mellitus type 2?
3) Which blood gas value would you expect to see in a client who has chronic obstructive pulmonary disorder?
4) Which blood gas value would you expect to see  in a client who has a pancreatic fistula and diarrhea?
5) Which blood gas value would you expect to see in a client 26 weeks pregnant with hyperemesis gravidarum?

*For NCLEX you do not have to worry about compensated or partially compensated blood gas interpretation.

# CHEST TUBES

A.) Chest tube is a _____ _____ drain that allow fluids or air to escape the pleural space

Remember normal breathing works on _____ _____.

Negative pressure is the idea that when humans inhale it is a result of the diaphragm contracting and moving down and the rib muscles move out. This causes the lungs to expand. The pressure inside the lungs drops. And it is the negative pressure that sucks the air in.

Chest tubes are needed whenever the _____ _____in the pleural space is disrupted.

Tension pneumothorax- _____is in between _____and _____which can be caused by trauma, surgery, falls etc. Outside air creates a one way valve inside the lung.

Classic signs of a tension pneumothorax:

| Trachea deviation | Yes |
|---|---|
| | |
| | |
| | |
| | |
| | |

This is a medical emergency, client needs treatment right away!

Treatment of tension pneumothorax:

# CHEST TUBES

**B.) Chest tube Setup:** All chest tube systems have these three chambers

| Collection chamber | Water Seal | Suction Control |
|---|---|---|
| Purpose is to:<br><br>Notify primary healthcare provider<br><br>1.<br><br>2. | Purpose is to:<br><br>Allow a_____ to exist from pleural space during<br><br>_____<br><br>&<br><br>_____air to enter the pleural space during<br><br>_____.<br><br>Bubbling/Tidaling<br><br>Continuous<br><br>Intermittent | Amount of suction applied to the client.<br><br>Both water seal and suction control have water in them.<br><br>Bubbling/Tidaling<br><br>Continuous-<br><br>Intermittent- |

## C.) Care of a client with a chest tube

1) Assess client for:

2) Chest tubes should be placed _____ chest level.

3) Do not milk or strip chest tube without a doctor's order.

4) Daily _____ x-rays are needed to check _____ _____.

5) Clients will have an _____dressing at the insertion site.

6) Never clamp a chest tube without a M.D. order.

D.) Common NCLEX troubleshooting……

1. Noticed the water seal is broken

A. Place the distal end of the tube in 2 cm of sterile water.

2. Pulled the chest tube out

A. Use a _____ _____.

B. Cover the opening with an _____ _____.

C. _____ the dressing on _____ sides only so that you can allow:

**Critical Think:  What is the difference between a regular sterile dressing & occlusive dressing?**

3.  Complains of pain won't comply-medicated and have the client to cough and deep breath
    A.
    B.

For NCLEX you have at the bedside of a client with a chest tube.

    1.
    2.
    3.

**Critically Think Future Nurses**

1. What kind of lung sounds would the nurse expect to hear with a client who needs a chest tube? Select all that apply.

    1. Wheezes
    2. Crackles
    3. Stridor
    4. Diminished
    5. Pleural friction rub

2. When caring for a client with a chest tube what should the nurse do to evaluate the effectiveness of the chest tube?

    1.  Empty chest tube drainage every shift
    2.  Mark chest tube drainage every shift
    3.  Clamp the chest tube when transferring the patient
    4.  Add water to the water seal chamber when she notices it is low

3. What should be done once the fluid in the water seal chamber no longer fluctuates with inspiration or expiration?


4. After a client has his chest tube removed by the healthcare provider which dressing should the nurse have ready to place over the incision site?

    1. Transparent film dressing
    2. Xeroform petroleum dressing
    3. Seaweed healing dressing
    4. Sterile cotton dressing

# VENT ALARMS

| ReMar Tip about Ventilator Alarms | High alarm sound=<br><br>Caused by: mucous, blockage, biting |
| --- | --- |
| | Low alarm sound=<br><br>Caused by: |
| If you don't know what to do then: | Disconnect the client and manually resuscitate them. |

## H.O.L.D. Help

| H | High Alarm |
| --- | --- |
| O | Obstruction |
| L | Low Alarm |
| D | Disconnection |

# CONGESTIVE HEART FAILURE

When the _____ cannot pump enough blood and nutrients to meet the needs of the organs.

Big Problem:

| _____ Side | _____ Side |
|---|---|
| L think | R think |
| Signs: | Signs: |

Most clients will have failure _____ _____ _____.

## B.) Diagnostic Tests

## C.) Medications

1.

2.

3.

4.

## D.) Nursing Interventions

# CONGESTIVE HEART FAILURE PRACTICE QUESTIONS

1. Mr. Green is scheduled to receive furosemide 60 mg IV BID for a diagnosis of congestive heart failure. The medication will have which of the following effects? Select all that apply.

   1. Decrease blood pressure
   2. Increase urine output
   3. Increase blood pressure
   4. Decrease urine output
   5. Decrease pain
   6. Increase edema

2. A 62-years-old client presents with dyspnea and blue colored nails and lips. The client has a suspected history of congestive heart failure and is admitted to emergency room. The client has not been compliant with his medication regimen and states he has not taken his hydrochlorothiazide for 4 days. The nurse should anticipate a diagnosis of which of the following?

   1. Pneumonia
   2. Pulmonary edema
   3. Pneumothorax
   4. Atelectasis

3. You are teaching the parents of a child with congestive heart failure about fluid intake. Which statement indicates understanding of monitoring fluid retention?

   1. I will calculate all of the fluids that my child drinks as this is the best method to monitor fluid retention.
   2. I will weigh each diaper daily as this is the best way to monitor fluid retention.
   3. I will weigh the child each day at the same time as this is the best way to determine fluid retention.
   4. I will listen to the lungs with my stethoscope as this is the best way to monitor fluid retention.

4. A client comes into the wellness clinic after being diagnosed with congestive heart failure. She complains of becoming tired after only very little activity. Which activity suggestion would the nurse give to preserve energy and decrease oxygen demands?

   1. Setting a specific time during the day and accomplishing all daily tasks at one time.
   2. Eating small frequent meals throughout the day.
   3. Removing oxygen therapy during rest to build up a tolerance without it.
   4. Exercise shortly after waking up in the morning when energy levels are highest

# DIAGNOSTIC PROCEDURES

1. Lumbar puncture

Position:

Client Teaching:

2. _____ non-invasive test that uses _____ to

create a detailed picture.

Position:

Client Teaching:

3.

Position:

Client teaching:

4. Esophagogastroduodenoscopy

Position:

Client Teaching:

5.

Position:

Client teaching:

*Before exam:* Do not take anticoagulants and herbal medications.

*After exam: What is the most serious complication after a liver biopsy?*

# DIAGNOSTIC PROCEDURES

6.

Position:

Client Teaching:

---

7. Angiogram or Arteriogram (RN only topic)

Position:

Client education:

*Before Exam:*

Medications to hold: Metformin, anticoagulants

*After the exam:*

*1. Assess the:*

*2. Bedrest for _____ to _____ hours.*

*\*Note: Some references say hold Metformin 24-48 hours before diagnostic study requiring IV iodine contrast media.*

# LOWERING CHOLESTEROL

The goal of therapy is to lower _____  _____ and _____  _____.

## Why does cholesterol matter?

## Values to know:

- LDL(Bad) =

- HDL (Good)=

- Total Cholesterol=

- Triglycerides=

| Examples of Dyslipidemias: |
| --- |

- *Simvastatin*
- *Rosuvastatin*
- *Atorvastatin*

*Note: Drug name ends in: Statin*

Side effects of Statins:

What about the B3 vitamin *Niacin*?

Side effects of Niacin:

| **Tip: Avoid flushed face by giving aspirin 30 minutes before treatment.** |
| --- |

When your client is on a dyslipidemia assess them for?

## What are the three types: _____.  _____. _____.

Which organ is damaged due to free flowing muscle fibers?

How will the muscle tissue be excreted?

How to treat:

NCLEX teaching about lowering cholesterol:

Goal of Low Cholesterol diet:

Avoid:

Dairy foods such as  cheese, butter, ice cream, egg yolk

Foods to include: avocados- which help raise HDL and lower LDL

# PHYSIOLOGICAL ADAPTATION HOMEWORK EXAM

1. A client is experiencing hyperventilation while receiving treatment on a mechanical ventilator. The nurse should monitor the client for:

   A. Hypercapnia
   B. Respiratory acidosis
   C. Respiratory alkalosis
   D. Decreased respiratory rate

2. Which position would provide the greatest respiratory capacity during an episode of dyspnea?

   A. Sims' position
   B. Supine position
   C. Orthopneic position
   D. Semi-Fowler's position

3. A nurse is caring for a client diagnosed with acute pleuritis. Which of the following is the **most** important to include in the plan of care?

   A. Administer pain medication frequently
   B. Assess for signs of pneumonia
   C. Administer medications to reduce cough
   D. Restrict fluids to reduce pulmonary edema

4. A client has just returned from a bronchoscopy. Which of the following is the **best** way to assess the return of the gag reflex?

   A. Inserting a tongue depressor to the back of the throat.
   B. Asking the client to say 4 or 5 short words.
   C. Monitoring the client while swallowing 5 ml of water.
   D. Asking the client to cough and deep breathe.

5. A client is being discharged from the hospital to complete his tuberculosis treatment at the outpatient clinic. Which of the following diets should the nurse instruct the client to maintain?

   A. A liquid diet with protein supplements
   B. A low calorie, low protein diet
   C. A high calorie, low protein, high carbohydrates diet
   D. A high calorie diet with frequent small meals
   E. A low calorie, low dairy and low carbohydrates diet

6. A nurse is caring for a client 10 hours following a left pneumonectomy. The nurse should place the client in which position?

   A. Left side-lying or supine
   B. Right or left side-lying position
   C. High Fowler's or right side-lying
   D. Right side-lying or prone

7. A client with lung cell cancer is scheduled for biopsy. Which of the following should be included in the client education?

   A. Take your aspirin as normal.
   B. Eat nothing after midnight.
   C. You will require a chest tube to assist with the procedure.
   D. An iodine contrast may be used to visualize the location of the cancer.

8. A nurse is caring for a client scheduled for a thoracentesis. The nurse knows:

    A. A thoracentesis may increase respiratory distress immediately after the procedure.
    B. The thoracentesis is used to remove fluid and blood from the thoracic cavity.
    C. The thoracentesis may negatively affect the client's blood pressure.
    D. The thoracentesis is used to increase the circulating fluid volume.

9. A nurse is working in the post-operative unit. Which is the **most** important action to ensure adequate ventilation?

    A. Administer oxygen while the client is sedated.
    B. Assess the client's lung sounds per doctor's order.
    C. Obtain a pulse oximetry reading if oxygen saturation is less than 95%.
    D. Place the client in the lateral position with the neck extended.

10. A nurse is caring for a client with a chest tube. During ambulation, the client's chest tube becomes separated from the drainage system? Which of the following is the **best** action by the nurse?

    A. Clamp the chest tube.
    B. Place the client in a high Fowler's position.
    C. Reconnect the chest tube to the drainage system.
    D. Prepare the client for reintubation.

# PHYSIOLOGICAL ADAPTATION PROGRESS EXAM

1. A client who has a newly placed percutaneous endoscopic gastrotomy (PEG) tube is requesting a bed bath. Which instruction should be given to unlicensed assistive personnel (UAP)?

    A. Monitor the client for residuals over 500 mL.
    B. Report any redness around the tube insertion site.
    C. Evaluate the client's response to pain medication during the bath.
    D. Check the client's blood glucose level.

2. A nurse is caring for a 4-year-old with a diagnosis of congestive heart failure. Which of the following signs would indicate a decrease in cardiac output?

    A. Fever
    B. Increased urine output
    C. Hypertension
    D. Delayed capillary refill

3. The school nurse has received a report that a child in the third grade has been diagnosed with cardiac disease. Which of the following symptoms would support a diagnosis of congestive heart failure?

    A. Abdominal pain
    B. Inability to run short distances
    C. Muscle tremors
    D. Dilated pupils

4. A twenty-month-old child with congestive heart failure is scheduled to receive digoxin. The nurse should hold the medication if the apical pulse is:

    A. Greater than 60 bpm
    B. Less than 50 bpm
    C. Greater than 100 bpm
    D. Less than 100 bpm

5. A nurse is caring for an infant with a heart defect that has a result of left to right shunting. The nurse should expect which diagnosis?

  A.  Cardiopulmonary obstructive disease
  B.  Tetralogy of Fallot
  C.  Congestive heart failure
  D.  Atrial septal defect

6. A client presents to the emergency department with acute chest trauma and respiratory distress. Which assessments are of the highest priority?

  A.  Respiratory ventilation status and presence of pulses
  B.  Blood pressure and the presence of pulses
  C.  Level of consciousness and respiratory rate
  D.  Respiratory rate and blood pressure

7. A client with a displaced chest tube requires mechanical ventilation. When suctioning the endotracheal tube, the nurse should:

  A.  Hyper-oxygenate the client with 100% oxygen before and after suctioning
  B.  Suction up to four times only during the procedure to expel mucus
  C.  Use short thrusting motions to enter the sensitive respiratory passage
  D.  Apply suction while gently inserting the catheter

8. The nurse is caring for a client in respiratory distress. The client has early indications of respiratory acidosis, which include:

  A.  Bradypnea
  B.  Restlessness
  C.  Nausea
  D.  Clubbing of the fingers

9. When caring for a client with a chest tube, the nurse observes some skin elevation around the insertion site. When the area is palpated, the nurse hears crackles. How should the nurse document this finding?

  A.  Rales
  B.  Airway blockage
  C.  Pitting edema
  D.  Crepitus

10. A female client with lung cancer is scheduled for a biopsy. Which of the following should the nurse include in the client education?

  A.  This procedure is different from percutaneous needle aspiration.
  B.  You will need to remain NPO after midnight.
  C.  There will be fluid removed from your abdominal cavity during the procedure.
  D.  The procedure will allow the physician to visualize the lungs.

# EAR SPOTLIGHT

Meniere's Disease:  A _____ disease that occurs in the _____ear resulting in

too much endolymphatic _____.

Does Meniere's affect 1 ear or 2 ears?  _____.

**The cause of Meniere's is:**

3 main symptoms:

1. Vertigo
2.
3. Hearing _____ _____

The patient may also complain of:
Best position during a Meniere's attack:

Diagnosis:

**Diet:**

**Treatment:**

1. Medical
2. Surgical

**NCLEX Prep:**

**Avoid:**

# DIABETES OVERVIEW

A.) _____ _____ is a _____

_____ in which the _____ _____ levels

are too _____.

| Two types of Diabetes Mellitus | Diabetes Type 1 | Diabetes Type 2 |
|---|---|---|
| 1) Age | | |
| 2) Is body producing insulin? | | |
| 3) Insulin dependent | | |
| 4) Ketone production | | |
| 5) Treatment | | 1.<br>2.<br>3.<br>4. Oral Non-Insulin Medications |

**B.) Signs/Symptoms:**

# DIABETES OVERVIEW

**B.)**

1.

2.

3.

**C.) Complications of Diabetes.**          Normal blood glucose level is: _____

| Hyperglycemia | Diabetes Type 1 | Diabetes Type 2 |
|---|---|---|
| **Cause** | Diabetic Ketoacidosis (DKA) | Hyperosmolar, Hyperglycemic Non-Ketotic (HHNK) |
| **Signs** | A- Acidosis ph less than 7.30 | |
| **Treatment** | Which IV fluid is best, dextrose water or 0.9% Sodium chloride? | |

# DIABETES OVERVIEW

## D. ) Complications continued

| Hypoglycemia | Diabetes Type 1 | Diabetes Type 2 |
|---|---|---|
| **Cause** | 1.<br><br>2.<br><br>3.Excessive exercise | Insulin overdose<br><br>Too little food<br>Excessive exercise |
| **Signs** | 1. Feeling irritable | 1. Shock |
| **Treatment** | | |

*The practical nurse treatment for the unconscious client is glucagon via IM injection. The solution is clear. The normal dose is 1 mg for adults and 0.5 mg for children.

## Laboratory Value

1.) Hemoglobin A1C is a blood test used to determine blood sugar control over_____ months.

You want it to be less than _____.

E.)Insulin Types and Actions

| Types | Generic Name | Onset | Peak | Duration |
|---|---|---|---|---|
| **Rapid** | *Insulin Aspart* | | 1 hour | 3 hours |
| **Short acting** | | Give this 30-mins. before meal | | |
| **Intermediate Acting solutions** | | | | |
| **Long Acting** | Glargine Determir | | | When do you give glargine? <br><br> Can you mix with other insulins? <br><br> Do you shake this insulin? |
| **70/30 mixtures** <br><br> **70-Regular** <br> **30-NPH** | Human 70/30 Novolog 70/30 | 30 minutes | 2 hours | 12 hours |

# DIABETES OVERVIEW

**Anti-hyperglycemia Oral Agents**

| Medications | Side Effects | Client Education |
|---|---|---|
| **1.** _____<br><br>Class Biguanides | *B12 deficiency*<br><br><br>Rare side effect: Lactic acidosis | First treatment recommended.<br><br>Take with meals.<br><br>Decreases sugar/glucose production by the _____.<br>Can you take during pregnancy?<br><br>**NCLEX Pro Tip:**<br>Metformin can also be used for polycystic ovary syndrome. |
| **Sulfonylureas**<br><br><br>**Tolbutamide**<br>**Glyburide**<br>**Glipizide**<br>**Glimepiride**<br><br>**Class Sulfonylureas** | | 1.<br><br>2.<br><br>Can you take during pregnancy?<br><br>NCLEX ProTip:<br>Glyburide and Metformin can be taken together to control blood glucose levels. Clients will face side effects of both |

# RN TEACHING SECTION NOTES

1.

2.

Vomiting after taking PO medications?

3.

4.

5.

6.

# DIABETES OVERVIEW

## Clinical Judgement Questions

1. A client with type 2 diabetes mellitus is scheduled for hip surgery in 12 hours. The client is currently NPO. The healthcare providers writes an order to continue home medications. The client takes metformin PO in the mornings. Which is the **most** appropriate intervention by the registered nurse?

    1. Call the healthcare provider to request a snack to be given in the morning.
    2. Give the morning medication after pharmacy sends it up to the unit.
    3. Call the healthcare provider and clarify the metformin order.
    4. Give IV insulin to regulate the blood glucose levels.

2. A client has received discharge teaching about insulin and a diabetes mellitus type II diagnosis. Which of the following is the **most** important teaching point for the registered nurse to begin with?

    1. Asking the patient to demonstrate how to measure and administer insulin.
    2. Explaining ways of storing insulin and utilizing syringes.
    3. Giving information on how many calories are needed with each meal.
    4. Teaching about the long term side effects of poor insulin control.

3. A six-years-old boy is taken to the emergency department with lethargy. The boy has diabetes mellitus. He appears to be dehydrated—his eyes are sunken and mucous membranes are dry. He has a two week history of polydipsia, polyuria, and weight loss. Which blood gas value would you expect?

    1. respiratory acidosis
    2. respiratory alkalosis
    3. metabolic acidosis
    4. metabolic alkalosis

# DIABETES OVERVIEW

---

**Advanced Clinical Topics: External Insulin Pumps**

---

1. _____ insulin pumps are _____ operated devices for

type _____ and _____ _____diabetes mellitus.

2. Insulin pumps use _____ or _____ action insulins.

3. Insulin pumps have soft _____ _____ inserted under the skin.

## Advantages:

No need for _____ _____.

Client can program the insulin pump to deliver a specific amount of _____.

Insulin pump can give _____ and bolus doses.

Pumps keep _____of the insulin administered.

## Disadvantages:

Skin irritations are _____.

Wearing the pump is a constant reminder of the _____.

Pump can be expensive.

## Question:

Does the client still need to check their blood glucose levels?

Does the client need to rotate the pump insertion site?

Can a client with an insulin pump have an MRI?

# ENDOCRINE REVIEW

**Thyroid hormones helps to regulate:**

| Hyperthyroidism | Hypothyroidism |
|---|---|
| *Signs:* <br><br> High _____ <br> High _____ <br> Heat _____ <br><br><br> Also called: Graves disease | Signs: |
| *Treatment:* <br> Diet: <br><br> Option 1: Radioactive iodine therapy <br><br> *Precautions:* <br><br><br> Visitors less than 1 hours. <br> No pregnant or nursing mothers to care for client. <br><br> Or <br><br> Option 2: Thyroidectomy | *Treatment:* <br><br> *Diet:* <br><br> *Hormone replacement* |

| | |
|---|---|
| *Thyroid Emergency:* Thyroid storm | *Watch For:* |
| | *Nursing Care:* |
| Treatment: | |
| *Nursing Care after a thyroidectomy:*<br>*Could be partial or complete<br>thyroidectomy | |
| After a thyroidectomy is a hoarse voice normal? | |
| Frequent swallowing? | |
| Sore throat? | |
| Always keep | |

# ENDOCRINE REVIEW

---

**Adrenal Disorders**

---

**The adrenal glands are located:**

**The adrenal glands help us:**

1) Addison's disease is too little by the adrenal cortex

**Signs of Addison's:**

Lab profile

**Client with Addison have a decreased:**

**Treatment:**

2) Cushing's Syndrome "too much" by adrenal cortex.

**Signs/symptoms:**

Lab profile

**Treatment:**

(Remember never abruptly stop taking steroids teach client to taper the drug off)

# PHYSIOLOGICAL ADAPTATION PROGRESS EXAM

1. A client is prescribed glyburide. The client asks the nurse how the medication is helping their type 2 diabetes mellitus. The **best** response by the nurse is which of the following?

    A. It increases the production of beta cells.
    B. It stimulates the release of insulin by the beta cells.
    C. It Increases insulin by the liver as an alternative.
    D. It increases the release of stored glycogen in the fat cells.

2. The healthcare provider orders 30 units of insulin to be added to 250 mL of normal saline. The nurse understands the only insulin to prepare is which of the following?

    A. Humulin N insulin
    B. Humulin R insulin
    C. Insulin Aspart
    D. Determir

3. A client is prescribed glipizide. Which of the following is the **most** important topic to educate the client on:

    A. Ketoacidosis
    B. Hypoglycemia
    C. Weight loss
    D. Dehydration

4. The nurse is aware the client with diabetes mellitus type 1 has understood the client education when he makes which of the following statements?

    A. I will drink orange juice to increase my blood glucose levels when I feel shaky and tired.
    B. I will drink orange juice to increase my blood glucose levels when I feel abdominal pain.
    C. I will drink orange juice to increase my blood glucose levels when I am thirsty and have headaches.
    D. I will drink orange juice with my breakfast to keep my blood glucose levels in a normal range.

5. A client has been prescribed propylthiouracil (PTU). Which of the following statements should be included in the client education?

    A. This medication will be taken for the rest of your life.
    B. This medication should be taken with meals.
    C. This medication will take effect within the first few weeks.
    D. This medication is best used in clients less than 250.

6. A nurse is caring for a client with diabetes insipidus. Which medication should he prepare to administer?

    A. Vasopressin
    B. Furosemide
    C. Regular insulin
    D. Intravenous fluids
    E. 5% Dextrose

7. Which of the following assessment findings characterize thyroid storm?

    A. Increased body temperature, decreased pulse, and increased blood pressure.
    B. Increased body temperature, increased pulse, and increased blood pressure.
    C. Increased body temperature, decreased pulse, and decreased blood pressure.
    D. Increased body temperature, increased pulse, and decreased blood pressure.

8. A nurse educator is teaching a conference about diabetes mellitus. A licensed practical nurse asks the educator to explain diabetes mellitus type II. Which of the following statements should the nurse include in her education?

    A. "With type 2 diabetes, the client is dependent on an outside source of insulin."
    B. "With type 2 diabetes, the body of the pancreas becomes inflamed."
    C. 'With type 2 diabetes, insulin secretion is decreased and insulin resistance is increased."
    D. "With type 2 diabetes, the body produces auto antibodies that destroy b-cells in the pancreas."


9. The pancreatic beta cell secrete the _____ hormone.


10. Which electrolyte does aldosterone directly regulate the concentration of? _____


# CLINICAL JUDGEMENT ACTIVITY #12
## "NCLEX NEXT-GEN STYLE QUESTIONS"

From the following terms in the box complete the paragraph about hyperthyroidism.

| | | |
|---|---|---|
| antibodies | exophthalmos | hypoventilation |
| bradycardia | goiter | neoplastic |
| cancer cells | polydactyly | tachycardia |
| hyperventilation | hypersecretion | thyroid |

Hyperthyroidism is also known as thyrotoxicosis. It is marked by an excess of 1. _____

hormones. Many consider it to be an autoimmune disorder caused by

2. _____ that bind to the thyroid gland cells and cause a 3. _____ of

hormones such as T3 triiodothyronine and T4 thyroxine. This will cause the client to have an enlarged thyroid gland,

called 4._____. An abnormal protrusion of the eyes is called 5. _____. Other clinical

symptoms include weight loss, sweating, restlessness, insomnia, rapid heartbeat or 6. _____.

| Answer box.    1. Thyroid    2. Antibodies.    3. Hypersecretion.    4. Goiter.    5. Exophthalmos    6. Tachycardia |
|---|

# THERAPEUTIC COMMUNICATION

The purpose of using these strategies is to help your client express their feelings more effectively.

S. Sit in _____

O. _____ with openness

L. Listen and lean forward

A. _____ eye level

R. _____ and rephrase

## Don't Do This:

Giving _____opinions

_____ the subject

_____ reassurance

_____with the client

Use words like bad, good, wrong or right

On NCLEX Choose......

1.

2. Never promise:

## Look for:

1. Open ended _____

2. Answers that focus on feelings

3. Answers that _____

Therapeutic communication allows clients to make their own choices

# THERAPEUTIC COMMUNICATION

**_____ Parameters**

| Age | Hold |
|-----|------|
|  | Less than |
|  | Less than |
|  | Less than |
|  | Less than |

## IMPORTANT Drug Antidotes

| Medication | Antidote |
|-----------|----------|
| Magnesium Sulfate | Calcium gluconate |
| Insulin |  |
|  | Protamine sulfate |
|  |  |
|  | Vitamin K, Fresh frozen plasma |

## Needle Information

| Route | Skin layers | Gauge | Length |
|-------|-------------|-------|--------|
| **SQ** | Epidermis, dermis and into the subcutaneous fat |  |  |
| **Intradermal** |  |  |  |
| **Intramuscular** |  | 22 | 1 Inch |

# PSYCHOLOGICAL CONCEPTS

1.

_____ is an acute _____ change that

is reversible with _____.

**Causes:**

| | |
|---|---|
| S | |
| I | |
| D | |
| E | |

**Assessment note:** Client will have a decreased level of consciousness.

**Memory Impairment Note**: Client will have a decreased short term memory

**Treatment:**

---
**NCLEX Point:** Research shows that even experienced nurses confuse the symptoms of delirium with dementia.
---

2. Dementia

Dementia is a _____ progressive

_____ _____ that has no cure. The disease also affects

    1.

    2.

    3.

The most common form of dementia is _____.

**Critically Think**

**Is Alzheimer's disease considered a mental illness?**

---
**Know the** _____ **of Alzheimer's Disease and also find these in Quick Facts**
---

1._____- inability to use an object correctly, client is unable to recognize what it is for.

2. Alexia-

3._____- inability to communicate

4. _____

## 3. Stages of Alzheimer's

| 1. Mild/Early | |
| --- | --- |
| 2. | A's<br>Agnosia<br>Alexia<br>Aphasia<br>Apraxia |
| 3. Severe/ Late | Incontinence of bowel and bladder<br><br>Further decline in cognitive and psychomotor coordination. |

# PSYCHOLOGICAL CONCEPTS

**Treatment**

_____ and _____ should be provided by the nurse.

When _____ is not appropriate then

_____ is the next action.

| NCLEX Tips: Other Nursing Interventions |
| --- |
| 1. Maintain a strict schedule to promote a sense of security<br>2. Keep a calendar/clock in sight.<br>3. Keep familiar objects such as family photos and objects from the past in the client's environment.<br>4. Address the client's caregivers to provide support. |

**4.** _____

These clients are _____ to _____.

| | Depression = Extreme Sadness | Mania = Extreme elation |
| --- | --- | --- |
| **Signs** | *all signs are negative*<br><br>No pleasure in things<br><br>Crying<br><br><br>Suicidal Thoughts | *all signs are positive*<br><br>Impulsive<br><br>Pleasure seeking |
| **Similarities** | | |
| **Treatments**<br>**The treatment is the same for both.** | Laboratory test: | Mood stabilizers, Counseling, lithium antipsychotics |

**Critically think: Circle the diagnosis based on the symptom.**

| | | |
|---|---|---|
| 1. Difficulty accepting compliments | Depression | Mania |
| 2. Bizarre dress | Depression | Mania |
| 3. Euphoria | Depression | Mania |
| 4. Fear | Depression | Mania |
| 5. Impulsiveness | Depression | Mania |

| | |
|---|---|
| **NCLEX Safety Point** | **Depression:**<br><br>**Nursing Interventions:** |
| | **Mania:** Defensive and against authority |

**5.** _____ - can't tell the difference

between _____ and _____.

Disease is _____ and requires _____treatment.

**Positive Psychotic Symptoms**

1. **Delusions-**

2. **Hallucinations-**

3. **Neologism-**

4. **Echolalia- constantly repeating something they heard**

5. **Flight of Idea- jumping from topic to topic during conversation**

**Negative Signs**: mute catatonic, suicidal, homicidal

**Treatment:**

**Medical:** Antipsychotic medications

**Environmental:** Nurse behavior

**Use** _____

**Sit in silence**

**Set** _____

# PSYCHOLOGICAL CONCEPTS

**Nursing Care:**

1. Always keep in mind _____.

2. _____their _____.

3. Present _____.

4. Set _____.

5. Avoid _____ the _____.

# PSYCH MEDICATIONS

1.) _____ - are used to reduce anxiety

**Medication Examples**

1.

2.

3.

4.

    1. _____ term use only.

    2. _____

    3. Safer to use in elderly than typical anti-psychotic medication

    4. Monitor clients with: _____.

    5. Monitor ataxia, liver function, and bone marrow suppression.

**Benzodiazepines can also be used as:**

    1.

    2.

    3.

    4. Treatment for alcohol withdrawal symptoms

**Side Effects:**

> **A-**

> **B-**

**Constipation, Confusion**

**Dry mouth**

**Sedation**

**Stasis of urine**


**-If clients overdose on benzodiazepines give?**

| Client Education Points Self-Reading Activity | 1. Give at bedtime. 2. Teach clients do not mix with alcohol. 3. Gradually taper off medication do not stop abruptly. |
|---|---|

2._____.

_____ is used to treat insomnia.

**Points to know:**

Treatment is short term and should last _____days.

Side Effects:

| Client Education Points | 1. Give immediately before bed 2. Can be given with food but for best effect take on empty stomach. |
|---|---|

| **Antipsychotic Medication** |
|---|
| 1. 2. |

# PSYCH MEDICATIONS

**Typical Antipsychotics**

**Two Types:**

**1.) Phenothiazines-**

**Examples:**

**Route:**

Side Effects: ABCDS + _____    _____

**Note: Tardive dyskinesia is considered an extrapyramidal effect.**

**Nursing Assessments:**

1. Monitor for _____ _____.
2. Monitor _____ _____especially temperature.
3. Teach clients to lay flat for _____ after administration.
4. Monitor for _____ _____.
5. Phenothiazines takes _____ _____to begin working.

**2. )Non-phenothiazine**

**Monitor client for:**

_____ + _____

**What drug can we give to lessen side effects?**  Benztropine

We have to tell patients that: Side effects are normal and expected. They have to keep taking drugs or the psychotic symptoms will return.

| NCLEX Psych Emergency |
|---|

_____ - an adverse reaction to anti-psychotic drugs.

Signs: _____ + _____ + _____

Nursing Care:

_____ - also used to treat psychotic symptoms but newer medications

**Examples:**

Atypical antipsychotics have less extrapyramidal symptoms

Monitor your patient for _____     _____.

**Atypical antipsychotics can cause:**

    1)

    2)

    3)

**NCLEX Pro-Tip:** Typical Psych medications can also be called:

**Atypical Psych medications can also be called:**

| NCLEX Psych Emergency |
|:---:|

_____ -

**Signs:**

**Nursing Care:**

**2.) Antidepressants**

1. _____

These drugs block M.A.O. enzyme that breaks down epinephrine, dopamine, and serotonin which leads to depression. They also block tyramine which puts clients at risk for a hypertensive crisis.

***MAOI's are not used as often due to various drug and food interactions***

**Examples:**

    1.

    2.

    3.

    4.

**Side Effects:** ABCDS is seen in vital sign changes along with INSOMNIA

**Diet Restrictions:** See Tyramine diet chart

**Client Teaching:**

        Medication may take 4-6 weeks to work.

        Never give MAOI's with Tricyclics or SSRIs

# PSYCH MEDICATIONS

**Tyramine Restricted Diet**

| Meats | |
|---|---|
| Grains | |
| Fruits | |
| Vegetables | |
| Dairy | |
| Sweets/Oils | |
| Condiments | |

**Antidepressants**

2. _____

These drugs inhibit the reuptake of serotonin in the treatment of depression

| Medication | Teaching |
|---|---|
| Fluoxetine | |
| | |
| | |
| | |

**Contraindications:**

**Client Teaching:**

1) St. John's Wort-


2) All S.S.R.I. may cause SAD head if too much is taken.


**Symptoms:**          **S**

                                **A**

                                **D**

                                **Head**


3. _____also used to treat depression also increases serotonin, and norepinephrine

**Examples:**

     1.

     2.

     3.
     4. Imipramine
     5. Clomipramine


TCAs can be used for childhood: enuresis


**Side Effects of TCAs:**

Cardiac changes: Tachycardia, orthostatic hypotension EKG changes
(Example long QT intervals)

**Client education:**
     1.

     2. Do not consume _____

     3. May take _____ _____ to achieve therapeutic levels.

     4. Take medication appropriately:

# PSYCHOSOCIAL INTEGRITY HOMEWORK EXAM

1. A client is taking sertraline for depression. The client has been taking the medication for two weeks and develops a urinary tract infection. The healthcare provider orders azithromycin to treat the disease. Which action should the nurse take?

    A. Notify the healthcare provider to discuss an alternative to azithromycin.
    B. Administer the medication as this combination is safe.
    C. Request an order to reduce the amount of sertraline.
    D. Request sertraline be stopped during antibiotic therapy.

2. The nurse is caring for a 26-years-old female client who is scheduled to receive a beta agonist. Before the administration of this medication, which assessment finding would **most** concern the nurse?

    A. A Respiratory rate of 27 breaths per minute.
    B. A heart rate of 115 beats per minute.
    C. A blood pressure of 100/60 mm Hg.
    D. A pulse oximetry reading of 92%.

3. A nurse is caring for a client diagnosed with schizophrenia. The client states, "Everyone is trying to poison my food!" Which is the **most** therapeutic response by the nurse?

    A.1. Why would the hospital staff poison the food?
    B. 2. You do not need to worry about poison, every medication I administer I will explain.
    C. 3. There is nothing to be afraid of.
    D. 4. You are in the hospital and you are safe.

4. The nurse is caring for a client with a history of alcohol abuse. Which of the following medications will prevent withdrawal symptoms?

    A. Chlorpromazine
    B. Lorazepam
    C. Terbutaline
    D. Phenobarbital

5. A client with bipolar disorder has been taking lithium and develops hypothyroidism. What will the nurse expect the physician to order for this client?

    A. Levothyroxine
    B. Lamotrigine
    C. Carbamazepine
    D. Cytochrome P450 enzymes

6. A nurse is working on a psychiatric unit. A client taking an MAOI is seen in the clinic with a blood pressure of 180/99 mm Hg. Which is the **most** important question for the nurse to ask the client?

    A. To describe the foods, the client ate that day.
    B. To inquire about grapefruit juice in the diet.
    C. To ask the client if increased activity was performed.
    D. To ask the client when was the last time they had their vitamin D levels monitored.

7. A client has been taking a selective serotonin reuptake inhibitor (SSRIs) for depression for eight months and tells the physician that the medication has not helped with symptoms. The provider plans to switch the client to an MAOI. The nurse should expect:

    A. The client will stop taking the SSRI and wait two weeks before taking the MAOI.
    B. The client will stop taking the SSRI and wait eight weeks before taking the MAOI.
    C. The client will begin taking the MAOI and stop taking the SSRI when the physician orders.
    D. The client will take both medications until symptoms are resolved.

8. An 18-years-old client in her senior year of high school is having anxiety about her graduation process. The client is diagnosed with an anxiety disorder. Which of the following is the **priority** treatment goal?

    A. The client will ask for her prescribed medication at the appropriate time.
    B. The client will sleep through the night.
    C. The client will describe ways to cope with anxiety.
    D. The client will not lose any weight during her treatment.

9. A client with a moderate level of anxiety is having an episode during her afternoon therapy session. Which medication would the psychiatrist **most** likely prescribe?

    A. Alprazolam
    B. Escitalopram
    C. Fluoxetine
    D. Sertraline

10. A nurse is caring for an elderly client with dementia. The client was found lying in the sun for 6 hours. The client is confused and unable to answer questions about his past medical history. Which nursing action is the **highest** priority?

    A. Contact the nearest family member to complete the medical history report.
    B. Assess the client's physical needs.
    C. Evaluate the client's mental needs.
    D. Contact the dietician to arrange a meal.

# PSYCHOSOCIAL INTEGRITY PROGRESS EXAM

1. The client asks a nurse, "What do you think about my new diagnosis?" The nurse replies, "What do you think about your new diagnosis?" The nurse is using which therapeutic communication technique?

    A. False Reassurance
    B. Reflecting
    C. Regression
    D. Acknowledgment

2. A nurse is caring for a client who was raped on the local college campus. The client is crying while describing the event to the nurse and social worker. Which response by the nurse is **most** appropriate?

    A. Medicate the client with a sedative.
    B. Arrange for the psychiatric healthcare provider to speak with the client.
    C. Listen quietly while the client continues to talk.
    D. Ask the client if she would like to discuss the event at another time.

3. A nurse is conducting a group therapy session; a 12-year-old male bipolar client becomes verbally abusive to the other participants. Which response is **most** therapeutic by the nurse?

    A. "If you do not sit down, you will be asked to leave the group."
    B. "You are misbehaving and causing a disruption. Please leave the group and go to your room."
    C. "Your behavior is inappropriate, let's go for a walk together to discuss what is happening."
    D. "If you are feeling upset, try to take a deep breath and calm yourself down."

4. A client is prescribed alprazolam. Which of the following is the **most** important statement to include in the client's education?

    A. Weekly group therapy sessions will be required while taking this medication.
    B. This medication must be taken with meals.
    C. Prolonged use of the medication could lead to addiction.
    D. This medication will reduce symptoms of bipolar disorder.

5. A nurse knocks on the door of a 19-year-old client diagnosed with paranoia. She enters the room without waiting and finds the client to be masturbating. The nurse should:

    A. Ask the client why he feels the need to masturbate
    B. Say excuse me and come back later
    C. Inform the client that it is time for his medication
    D. Ask the client if he needs privacy

6. A nurse is caring for a client diagnosed with schizophrenia. While assessing the hallucinations, the nurse is aware the **most** common type of hallucination is:

    A. Visual
    B. Olfactory
    C. Tactile
    D. Auditory

7. A client with schizophrenia refuses to attend a group therapy session. Which is the **best** response by the nurse?

    A. Inform the client that the therapy session will be helpful
    B. Allow the client to skip the therapy session
    C. Have the nurse manager approach the client about the required attendance
    D. Bring the group therapy session to the client's location

8. A nurse has administered clonazepam to a client, and fifteen minutes later the client presents with diplopia, impaired balance, and a rigid jaw. The nurse should expect to administer:

    A. Chlordiazepoxide
    B. Clorazepate
    C. Benztropine
    D. Thioridazine

9. Which of the following laboratory results are the **most** important before administering lithium?

    A. Fasting glucose tolerance exam
    B. Neurologic studies
    C. Glomerular filtration rate
    D. Pulmonary function test

10. Which of the following is associated with schizophrenia?

    A. Weight loss
    B. Sexual promiscuity
    C. Impetigo
    D. Disorganized speech

# CLINICAL JUDGEMENT ACTIVITY #13

**Based on the defintion determine which mental condition your client is suffering from.**

**ANSWER Choices:**

| | | | |
|---|---|---|---|
| Agoraphobia | Somatization disorder | Panic disorder | Schizophrenia |
| Anorexia nervosa | Social phobia | Bulimia nervosa | Bipolar disorder |

*A psychiatric condition where the client has an unstable mood pattern involving shifts from mania to depression.*
This client has_____.

*A mental disorder where the client has a deficit in thought processes and can be out of touch with reality.*
This client has _____.

*An excessive intake of calories followedd by self induced purging activities to avoid weight gain.*
This client has _____.

This disorder is accompanied with anxiety and repeated episodes of fear.
This client has _____.

The fear of public humiliation or acting in an embarrassing manner in front of people.
This client has _____.

A person who complains of many physical symptoms but no medical cause can be found.
This client has _____.

An extreme dieting and weight loss illness to the point of emaciation and potentially death.
This client has _____.

Attacks of fear where a person thinks they will be confined to a place with no way to escape.
This client has _____.

ANSWER KEY:
A. Bipolar disorder      B. Schizophrenia      C. Bulimia nervosa      D. Panic disorder
E. Social phobia      F. Somatization disorder      G. Anorexia nervosa   H.Agoraphobia

# ECG OVERVIEW

**Depolarization or Repolarization?**

_____

**What does it mean?** _____

**Why do we need to know it?** _____

     1. Start with the word _____

     2. When something is "polarized" it means:

There are special cells in the heart that generate electrical activity.

Electrical Activity Starts in the Sinus Node located in Right Atrium.

Depolarization means-

Ions move through channels. The 3 channels are:

     A.

     B.

     C.

**Movement of ions across cell membrane causes:**

Repolarization means-

During repolarization cardiac muscles are relaxed.

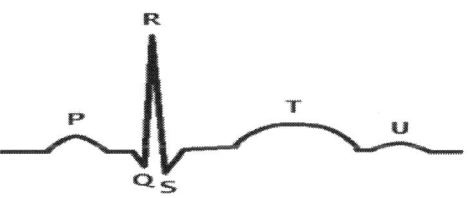

| Parts of the ECG | What is happening? |
|---|---|
| P wave | |
| | atrial repolarization and relaxation |
| | Ventricular repolarization and relaxation |
| | |

Note: EKG/ECG only shows you electrical activity not muscular activity.

## 1. Normal Sinus Rhythm

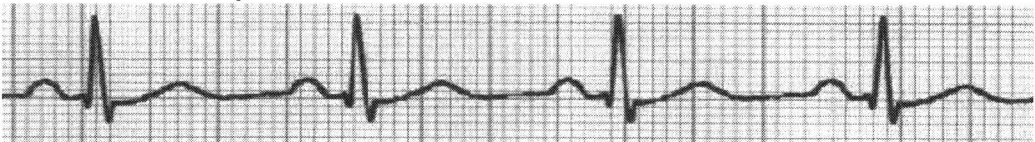

Can you circle each p wave on this ECG strip?

Can you circle each QRS complex on this ECG strip?

**Normal sinus rhythm =**

| | |
|---|---|
| **1. What is the rate?** | |
| **2. What is the rhythm?** | |
| **3. Is there a P wave before each QRS?** | |
| **4. Are the P waves upright and similar?** | |
| **5. What is the length of the PR interval?** | |
| **6. What is the length of the QRS complex?** | |

**Rules:** _____

**2.** _____

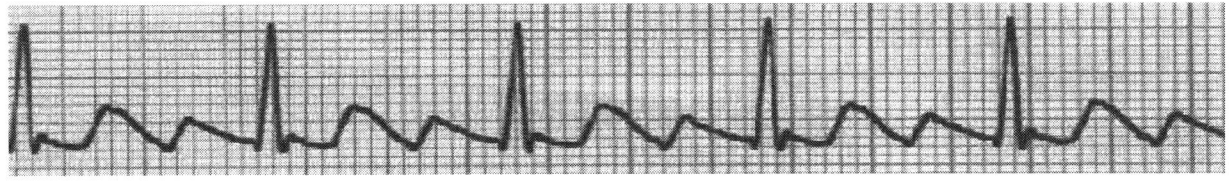

_____ = _____

| | |
|---|---|
| 1. What is the rate? | Atrial: 250-400 bpm<br>Ventricular: variable |
| 2. What is the rhythm? | Atrial: regular<br>Ventricular: irregular |
| 3. Is there a P wave before each QRS? | Normal P waves are absent |
| 4. Are the P waves upright and similar? | |
| 5. What is the length of the PR interval? | |
| 6. What is the length of the QRS complexes | 0.06-0.12 |

**These NCLEX patients have Atrial Flutter:**

| | | |
|---|---|---|
| Valve disorder (mitral) | Thickening of the heart muscle | Ischemia |
| Cardiomyopathy | COPD | Emphysema |

**NURSING INTERVENTIONS FOR ATRIAL FLUTTER**

_____ – treatment of choice for NCLEX!!!

**Slow the ventricular rate by using: diltiazem, verapamil, digitalis, or beta blocker.

Heparin to reduce incidence of thrombus formation.

**3.** _____

**Ventricular Tachycardia =**

| 1. What is the rate? | Atrial: Q<br>Ventricular: 100-200 |
|---|---|
| 2. What is the rhythm? | Regular |
| 3. Is there a P wave before each QRS? | Absent |
| 4. Are the P waves upright and similar? | Absent |
| 5. What is the length of the PR interval? | Not measurable |
| 6. What is the length of the QRS complexes | Wide greater than 0.12 sec |

**Assess first if the client is:**

**Stable =**

**Unstable =**

**These patients have ventricular tachycardia:**

Cocaine users          Chest trauma          DIGOXIN takers      Enlarged heart hx

Hypokalemia or low serum potassium

Treatment:

Never pick _____ as a treatment for

ventricular tachycardia because it:

What's the difference?

| C | |
|---|---|
| D | |

# EKG OVERVIEW

4. _____

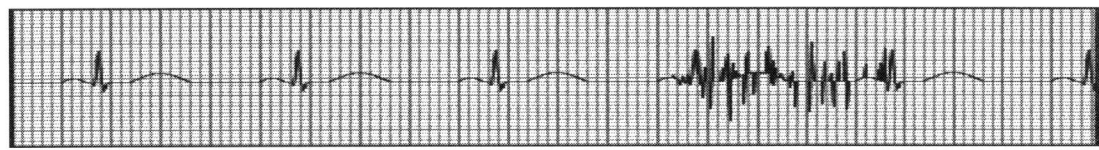

**Asystole =**

**Treatment:**

*If the monitor says asystole but the patient is clearly alive then check for electrode placement

5. _____

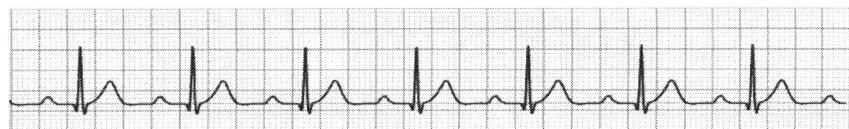

**Artifact-**

Do not put electrodes over hairy areas or bony prominences

**Possible causes are:**

Loose _____

Muscle _____

Client _____

**Treatment:**

**NCLEX Advanced Topics: Heart Blocks**

**First Degree Heart Block**

The PR interval is _____.

**Is this an emergency?**

What is the treatment?

What medications can cause first degree heart block?

# EKG OVERVIEW

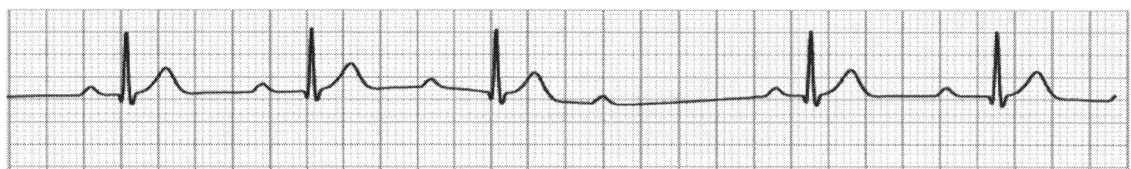

**Second degree heart block type 1 (Mobitz Type 1 or Wenckebach)**

The PR interval is _____, _____and then the _____ drops.

    Is this an emergency?

    What is the treatment?

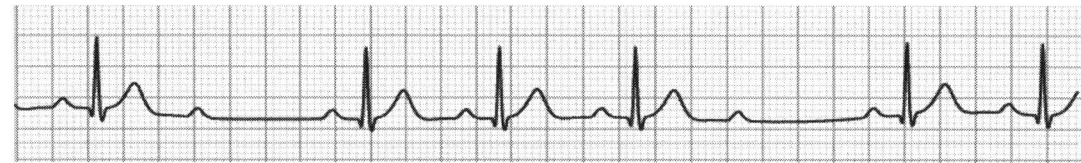

**Second degree heart block type 2 (Mobitz Type 2)**

The PR interval is _____ _____ and then the _____ _____ drops.

    Is this an emergency?

    What is the treatment?

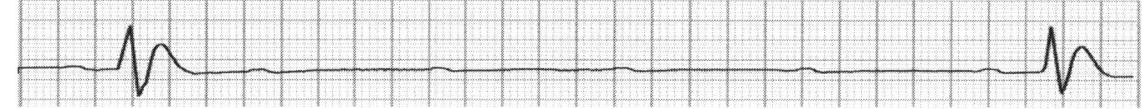

**Third degree heart block**

The _____ and _____ are beating _____ from _____ _____.

    Is this an emergency?

    What is the treatment?

**Critical Thinking Question.**

A registered nurse is caring for a client on continuous electronic heart monitoring. The client's electrical heart rhythm displays a progressively longer PR duration with a non-conducted p wave. Which type of heart block should the nurse document?

    1. First degree heart block
    2. Second degree, type 1
    3. Second degree, type 2
    4. Third degree

# ISOLATION PRECAUTIONS

**A.) Universal Precautions**

| |
|---|
| 1. Wash Hands |
| Alcohol-based Hand sanitizer Notes: |
| Need to contain over _____ alcohol |
| Can use if hands are visibly soiled? |
| What about coughing into hand? |
| What about rinsing hands while sanitizer is still wet? |
| How much alcohol hand sanitizer is enough? |
| 2. |
| 3. |

**B.)**

| |
|---|
| |

**Contact Disease:** MRSA, VRE, C. difficle,

**C.) Droplet Precautions**

| |
|---|
| |
| |
| |

**Droplet Disease:**

Can the client's door stay open with Contact Precautions?

Can a client's door stay open with Droplet Precautions?

**D.)**

| | |
|---|---|
| | |
| | |
| | |

**Airborne Disease:**

Varicella can be replaced with disseminated herpes zoster or shingles.

Can the clients door stay open with airborne precautions?

**Cohort Tip:**

| Disease | Precaution |
|---|---|
| AIDS | |
| Vaginal Yeast Infection | |
| Diarrhea | |
| Mononucleosis or Epstein Barr Virus | |
| West Nile Virus-transmitted by mosquitoes | |
| Hepatitis C | |
| MRSA- staph infection | |
| C-difficile | |
| Rota virus | |
| Shigellosis | |
| Head Lice | |
| Epiglottitis | |
| Influenza (seasonal) | |
| Rubella (German Measles) | |
| Whooping Cough (Pertussis) | |
| Meningitis | |
| Varicella (Chicken Pox) | |
| Monkey Pox | |
| Rubeola (Measles) | |

Remember cohort client with same precaution

# ISOLATION PRACTICE QUESTIONS

1. A nurse manager reports for duty and has to evaluate each nurse's assignment. A nurse has a client with A.I.D.S. and the nurse manager is evaluating his care by the healthcare team. She should intervene when she sees which situation?

    1. A housekeeper cleans up spilled blood with a bleach solution.
    2. A nurse takes the client's blood pressure wearing a mask and gloves.
    3. A phlebotomist wears gloves to perform a blood draw.
    4. A nurse attendant allows visitors to enter his room without masks.

2. A 7-year-old client is being admitted to the pediatric unit. What personal protective equipment must be placed outside the room when the nurse sees the client is diagnosed with varicella?

    1. Gloves, disposable thermometer, private room, 6 fresh air exchanges per hour
    2. Goggles, respiratory mask, gown, private room, gloves
    3. Gown, private room, goggles, 6 fresh air exchanges per/hour, respiratory mask
    4. Private room, goggles, respiratory mask, gloves, face/eye shield

3. What isolation precaution would you use for cutaneous anthrax?

    1. Standard
    2. Droplet
    3. Contact
    4. Airborne

4. What isolation precaution would you use for rotovirus?

    1. Standard
    2. Droplet
    3. Contact
    4. Airborne

# CLINICAL JUDGEMENT ACTIVITY #14

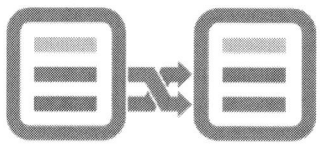

Match the condition with the associated organism.

| Condition | Organism |
|---|---|
| 1. Mononucleosis _____ | A. Blood borne hepatitis |
| 2. Hepatitis C _____ | B. Varicella zoster |
| 3. Gonorrhea _____ | C. Staphylococcus aureus |
| 4. Chicken pox _____ | D. Epstein-Barr virus |
| 5. Impetigo _____ | E. Neisseria gonorrhoaea |

Answer box
1. Mononucleosis is caused by Epstein-Barr virus. The virus is transmitted through saliva, but you can also get the virus by sharing drinks or utensils. The correct answer is D.
2. Hepatitis C is a viral infection that causes liver inflammation. It is spread by a blood borne hepatitis pathogen. The correct answer is A.
3. Gonorrhea is an infection caused by a sexually transmitted bacterium that infects both males and females. The correct answer is E.
4. Chicken pox is an infection caused by varicella zoster. The client will present with a red, itchy rash on the skin that covers the body. The correct answer is B.
5. Impetigo is a highly contagious skin infection that is common in infants and children. Impetigo usually appears as red sores around the nose, mouth, hands, and feet. The correct answer is C.

# ACCIDENT & ERROR PREVENTION

**1.**

**A.**

Why are children more at risk for medication errors?

Why do _____ work differently in _____?

1. Time of day
2.
3.

**B. Falls**

1.
2.
3.

**C.** S_____ E_____ - unanticipated _____

that happens in healthcare that results in the _____ or serious

_____ to a client.

**D**.

# ACCIDENT & ERROR PREVENTION

**Let's Talk Seizures:** Seizures start in the brain

1. Place _____ on the _____ side.

2. Do not _____ _____.

3. _____stimuli is _____.

4. Do not put _____ in the client's _____.

5. Keep _____ and _____ at the _____

## 2. Error Prevention

1. Restraints- are interventions used to reduce client harm.

2 Types: Chemical /Physical

## Can an RN put on a restraint without an order?

If there is no _____ or _____ restraints

are considered _____ _____.

_____ orders are called prescriptions.

## Prescriptions have

A.)

B.)

C.)

D.)

2. _____- Use _____ or _____ ink.

Writing is a legal document. It has to be _____.

_____ in charting-

3. _____ _____-form that details an unexpected event.

## Reasons to write:

1.
   *Do you assess the visitor?*

2.

3.

4.

# MANAGEMENT OF CARE

**\*Before watching the lecture. Study the definition box below.**

Registered nurses have  several responsibilities when a client is in need of care.
The registered nurse can functions such as a:

1. Staff Nurse-Responsible for several clients.
2. Charge Nurse-Responsible for a team of nurses and their quality of care.
3. Nurse Manager-Responsible for a team of nurses, their educational growth, policy and procedures and to monitor the daily budgets of a location.
4. Case Manager-assesses, plans, implements, and evaluates a client's health and social service needs.

**ReMar Pro-Tip:** Remember registered nurses have the responsibility of discharging a client and that conversation begins during the admission process.

_____ managers work directly with the _____ team.

_____ managers also _____ clients for _____ _____ and

connect clients to community resources.

**\*Case management is not managed care.**

\*Managed care are _____ used to lower or reduce the cost of _____ _____.

**Interdisciplinary Team**

The interdisciplinary team is a _____ group of _____ from

_____medical _____.

**The goal is to:**

     1. provide the _____ _____.

     2. reduce client _____.

     3. Reduce _____ stays

     4. Allow the client to have _____ of _____.

The teams come together at a multidisciplinary conference.

Which clients need multidisciplinary team?

The client with complex _____ _____.

_The role of the registered nurse on the interdisciplinary team is to:_

# CLINICAL JUDGEMENT ACTIVITY #15

Match the client with the most important disciplinary team member.

| | |
|---|---|
| 1. The 62-year-old-client diagnosed with a nasal gastric tube who has continuous diarrhea from the current formula. | A. Pharmacist |
| 2. A 4-year-old client admitted to the hospital for minor surgery who is afraid to have his temperature taken. | B. Speech therapist |
| 3. A 76-year-old elderly client who is taken several cardiac medications and is now diagnosed with seasonal influenza. | C. Occupational therapist |
| 4. A 14-year-old with back pain from a previous spinal surgery after a diagnosis of scoliosis. | D. Nutritionist |
| 5. An 8 year-old child resistant to speak in class due to a stutter. | E. Surgeon |
| 6. The 45-year-old client with multiple sclerosis who is unable to hold a spoon in her hand. | F. Registered Nurse |

# LEGAL ISSUES IN NURSING

A. Advanced Directives-_____ that allow clients to make decisions in _____.

They help to direct the client's _____ of _____.

| | 2. |
|---|---|
| DPA Notes<br><br>Person has to be 18 years or older. | Document that allows<br><br>to make decisions for<br><br>1.<br>2.<br>3. |

***Know client's _____status!!!

B) Informed Consent- _____ sure _____ is able to understand what is

going to happen during a procedure, exam, test.

| Need written consent to do | Can do without written consent |
|---|---|
| 1.<br>2. Administer Blood<br>3. Anesthesia | 1.<br><br>2. |

# LEGAL ISSUES IN NURSING

**Who responsibility is it?**

| |
|---|
| How to handle the Impaired (alcohol/alcohol abuse) nurse? |
| 1.    Get the facts, only report objective behaviors. Not your opinion. |
| 2.    Report to the supervisor or nurse manager. |
| 3.    Never confront the co-worker. |

**Clinical Judgement Scenarios:**

1. What if a client's attorney requests information?

2. What if the nurse is caring for a child and the parents are away can consent be obtained over the phone?

3. Can a client have a procedure done even though they refuse to sign a written consent?

# DELEGATION & ASSIGNMENT

What is the difference?

| |
|---|
| _____ is giving a specific _____ to a _____ who is capable of _____ the duty. When you _____ you still are _____. |

| |
|---|
| _____ is _____ a client's care or _____ to another provider. *When nurses receive assignments they have to take a report because* *they become responsible for that client's total care.* |

The nursing process _____.

## A. Delegation

| RN |
| --- |
| |

| LPN | Unlicensed Assistive Personnel or Aide |
| --- | --- |
| Stable client with routine care<br><br>Dressing changes (sterile)<br><br><br><br>*IV Piggyback secondary<br>Calculate IV flow rate<br><br><br>No: | Provide reassurance? |

# DELEGATION PRACTICE QUESTIONS

1. Who would be the most appropriate to feed a confused elderly client who can become combative?

    1.) RN
    2.) LPN/LVN
    3.) Nurse's Aide
    4.) Physical Therapist

2. Who would be most appropriate to assist a client ambulating down the hall for the first time after a hip replacement?

    1.) RN
    2.) LPN/LVN
    3.) Nurse's Aide
    4.) Speech Therapist

3. As part of the nurse's aide daily tasks she should complete the following tasks?
Select all that apply.

    1.) Bath the client _____
    2.) Provide assistance with ambulation_____
    3.) Chart and calculate intake for shift _____
    4.) Obtain sputum specimen _____
    5.) Assist with feeding _____

4. A nurse is caring for a client with increased intracranial pressure, the client suddenly becomes unresponsive. A code is called and the nurse calls for assistance, who is most appropriate to gather the code cart?

    1. Another registered nurse
    2. A licensed practical nurse
    3. A nurse's aide
    4. The charge nurse of the unit

# CLINICAL JUDGEMENT ACTIVITY #16

**Example A** - A charge nurse Jones assigns registered nurse Green to an unstable client who has cancer and high blood pressure for her shift. Nurse Green participates in a handoff report. The client does not receive safe or ethical medical care during the shift.

1. Who is responsible for the client's lack of safe ethical medical care? _____

**Example B** - An RN assigns a LPN to a stable and predictable client who is five days post-op a left knee replacement. The LPN fails to deliver competent care to the client by administering several wrong medications.

2. Who is responsible for the client's lack of competent medical care? _____

**Example C** - An LPN delegates an unlicensed care provider to take vital signs for clients in a progressive care setting. The nurse does not receive vital signs in proper time to prevent a hypotensive crisis. The client has to be transferred to the ICU as a result of lack of competent care.

3. Who is responsible to obtain the vital signs? _____

# CLINICAL JUDGEMENT ACTIVITY #17

Beside each listed nursing activity, circle who is most appropriate to complete the task.

|  | | | | |
|---|---|---|---|---|
| 1. Prepare a client for discharge | Aide | PN | RN | DR |
| 2. Discontinue a foley catheter | Aide | PN | RN | DR |
| 3. Insert a peripheral IV | Aide | PN | RN | DR |
| 4. Do range of motion on a patient in bed | Aide | PN | RN | DR |
| 5. Administer IM injections | Aide | PN | RN | DR |
| 6. Explain a diagnosis | Aide | PN | RN | DR |
| 7. Chart vital signs | Aide | PN | RN | DR |
| 8. Complete a sterile dressing change | Aide | PN | RN | DR |

|  | | | | |
|---|---|---|---|---|
| 9. Oral suctioning a client | Aide | PN | RN | DR |
| 10. Administering a bath to a terminally ill patient | Aide | PN | RN | DR |
| 11. Ambulating a client the first time after surgery | Aide | PN | RN | DR |
| 12. Follow-up teaching about a new medication | Aide | PN | RN | DR |
| 13. Obtaining a consent for xray | Aide | PN | RN | DR |
| 14. Transporting a stable client to xray | Aide | PN | RN | DR |

|  | | | | |
|---|---|---|---|---|
| 15. Irrigating a stage 4 infected wound | Aide | PN | RN | DR |
| 16. Obtain a hemoccult specimen | Aide | PN | RN | DR |
| 17. Triage clients | Aide | PN | RN | DR |
| 18. Administer pitocin to a women in labor | Aide | PN | RN | DR |
| 19. Insert a suprapubic catheter | Aide | PN | RN | DR |
| 20. Change a colostomy dressing | Aide | PN | RN | DR |
| 21. Chart urine output of a client with a foley | Aide | PN | RN | DR |
| 22. Feed a client with dysphagia | Aide | PN | RN | DR |

Answer Box

| | | | | | | | | |
|---|---|---|---|---|---|---|---|---|
| 1.RN | 2.PN | 3.RN | 4.Aide | 5.PN | 6.DR | 7.Aide | 8.PN | 9.PN |
| 10.Aide | 11.RN | 12.PN | 13.DR | 14.Aide | 15.PN | 16.PN | 17.RN | 18.RN |
| 19.DR. | 20.PN. | 21.Aide. | 22.RN | | | | | |

# PRIORITIZATION

All the answers will seem right but only one is the PRIORITY!

1.) A new nurse working in the emergency room department reports for duty. Four patients arrive at the same time, who should she see first?

> A. A 100-years-old female with a temperature of 102, chills, and diarrhea.
> B. A 55-years-old male with severe abdominal pain from a kidney stone.
> C. A 2-years-old female with a heat rash complaining of itching.
> D. An 89-years old female with a poor gag reflex.
> E. A client with a gunshot wound to the right upper extremity.

**Don't let NCLEX distract you with:** _____ **or** _____

**Only think about what is happening:**

**Look for the patient who is going to:**

## REVERSE PRIORITY

> 1. Least amount of _____
> 2. Least _____
> 3. Condition is plainly stated.

# PRIORITY PRACTICE QUESTIONS

1.) A nurse is working in the emergency department at your local hospital. Four patients approach the triage desk at the same time. List the order in which you will assess these clients.

> A. 50 years old female with moderate abdominal pain and occasional vomiting.
> B. A 9 years old irritable female with nuchal rigidity, petechiae, and a fever.
> C. A 22 years old jogger with a twisted ankle, having a pedal pulse and no bruising.
> D. A 19 years old male with a bandaged head wound.

2.) A nurse is working in the emergency department. She has 4 clients which should she see first?

> A. A 79-year-old female with her right arm in a sling. She states she was walking out to get her mail when she tripped on an uneven sidewalk and fell onto her right side. She denies hitting her head or losing consciousness. She has a positive radial pulse in the right arm, there is some deformity noted.
>
> B. A 53-year-old male holding his left hand with his right hand and states "I was working on my horse trailer, trying to connect the trailer to the truck when I dropped the hitch and it landed on my hand." Patient has a crushing injury to his 2nd and 3rd fingers on the left hand.
>
> C. A 67-year-old male with slurred speech and carrying a mason glass jar with a snake in it. He states he was drinking with his buddies when he saw a snake in the driveway. He was trying to catch it when it bit him on the right hand. The snake is a water moccasin.
>
> D. A 79 year old male brought to the ER from the nursing home after a fall. He stood up in his wheelchair without assistance and attempted to walk. He stumbled and fell onto his left side and did not hit his head or lose consciousness. There are no injuries present.

3.) These clients present to the ED complaining of acute abdominal pain. Prioritize them in order of severity.

> A. 22 years old college student complaining of severe, intermittent cramps with three episodes of watery diarrhea, 2 hours after eating.
>
> B. A 22 years old female with a low-grade fever, left lower quadrant tenderness, nausea and an inability to eat for the last 3 days.
>
> C. A 12 years old female with moderate left upper quadrant pain, vomiting small amounts of yellow bile, and worsening symptoms over the past 3 days.
>
> D. A 56 years old male with a pulsating abdominal mass and sudden onset of pressure-like pain in the abdomen and flank within the past hour.

# MANAGEMENT OF CARE HOMEWORK EXAM

1. Which nursing intervention is most appropriate immediately after the death of a client?

    A. Notifying the morgue unit
    B. Cleaning the body
    C. Contacting the next of kin
    D. Positioning the body to prevent post-death complications

2. A nurse is caring for a 90-year-old client diagnosed with pneumonia. Which symptoms would the nurse expect to see first?

    A. Sweating and fever
    B. Dyspnea and fever
    C. Chills and cough
    D. Dehydration and altered mental status

3. A nurse is conducting an educational session on anxiolytic medications. Which of the following is the priority statement to include?

    A. Notify the healthcare provider if drowsiness occurs.
    B. Do not take this medication with food.
    C. Avoid alcohol while taking this medication.
    D. Take the medication as needed for anxiety.

4. The nurse is assessing a client with suspected acute pancreatitis. Which finding is the most likely in the client's health history?

    A. Liver disease
    B. Congestive heart failure
    C. Diabetes mellitus
    D. Alcohol abuse

5. A nurse is working in a mental health clinic. During the client's history review, the client stands up in a chair and states, "I am a mailbox." Which of the following is the priority nursing statement?

    A. "You are not a mailbox and you will never be."
    B. "You do not need to pretend to be something you are not. There is no reason to be afraid."
    C. "There is no reason to act like this. No one is here to hurt you."
    D. "You are not a mailbox, you are a person. This is a hospital, and you are safe."

6. A nurse is working in the emergency room (ER). She has 4 clients, which should she assess first?

    A. A 79-year-old female arrives at the ER with her right arm in a sling. She states she was walking out to get her mail when she tripped on an uneven sidewalk and fell onto her right side. She denies hitting her head or losing consciousness. She has a positive radial pulse in the right arm, and there is some deformity noted.

    B. A 53-year-old male comes to the ER holding his left hand with his right hand and states, "I was working on my horse trailer, trying to connect the trailer to the truck when I dropped the hitch, and it landed on my hand." The patient has a crushing injury to his second and third fingers on the left hand.

    C. A 67-year-old male presents to the ER with slurred speech and carrying a mason glass jar with a snake in it. He states he was drinking with his buddies when he saw a snake in the driveway. He was trying to catch it when it bit him on the right hand. The snake is a water moccasin.

    D. A 79-year-old male is brought to the ER from the nursing home after a fall. He stood up in his wheelchair without assistance and attempted to walk. He stumbled and fell onto his left side and did not hit his head or lose consciousness. There are no injuries present.

7. A nurse has arrived on the scene of a tornado that collapsed an apartment building. Of the four clients lying in the parking lot, who should she treat first?

> A. A teenage girl trapped under an overturned piece of furniture. The only apparent injuries are scrapes, bruises, and a firm protrusion on her forehead. The respiration rate is 24 bpm, pulse 120 bpm, and strong with good capillary perfusion.

> B. A middle-aged male who is unconscious. There are large areas of blistered red burns on arms, chest, and face, with singed hair also on the face and head. Respirations are shallow, irregular, and very slow at 4-5 bpm.

> C. An infant girl about a year old, found under a dead victim. The infant cries loudly, moving arms and legs has blood on her, but with close examination, there is no evidence of injury. The child's clothes are soaked from water. No breathing distress noted, respirations are 28.

> D. A young woman who was found face down. There is a large bloody wound on the back of her head, with visible blood leaking through clothes in many spots. When rolled over, she is limp and completely unresponsive. When her eyes are open, one pupil is large and fixed. Breathing is slow and irregular at 14 beats per minute. Her pulse is 60 beats per minute.

8. There was a ruptured gas line and explosion at a large medical clinic. The registered nurse is assigned to triage. Which client should she see first?

> A. A school-aged boy standing in the middle of the room. Pale, shaking, and crying out loud. No obvious injuries.

> B. A teenage boy in shorts with blistered reddened skin covering both legs. No evidence of burns above the legs. The child is alert and talking but has severe pain and rates it ten on a scale of 0-10.

> C. A young woman, 37-weeks-pregnant who is reporting shortness of breath. The respiration rate is 38 bpm. They are shallow and strained. Skin pale, cool, and dry, with capillary perfusion greater than 2 seconds.

> D. A disheveled adult male who is poorly groomed. The client was found wandering around without purpose and mumbling. Some scratches and abrasions are noted, but no obvious injury. No breathing difficulties. He is able to identify his name and where he lives but his speech pattern is bizarre.

9. The nurse on a pediatric unit has received a report on four clients. The nurse should plan to assess which client first?

> A. A 3-years-old client with a temperature of 99.7 and a blood pressure of 70/45.
> B. A 5-years-old client with a history of asthma who has a peak expiratory flow rate of 83%.
> C. A 9-years-old with a fracture of the radial bone who is reporting pain rated 8 on a pain scale of 0 to 10.
> D. A 7-years-old client with ulcerative colitis who has had 16 blood tinged stools in the last 24 hours.

10. The nurse has received 4 clients from a house fire. Which client should she assessment first?

> A. The client who has the tibia bone protruding through the skin and is in severe pain.
> B. The client who has third-degree burns of the left foot and is crying.
> C. The client who is unconscious, pulseless, and has dilated pupils.
> D. The client who has soot on the face and the nares and is coughing.

# MANAGEMENT OF CARE PROGRESS EXAM

1. A nurse is caring for a client who is 6 hours post abdominal surgery. Which of the following interventions is the priority nursing action to prevent atelectasis?

    A. Reducing the client's pain with prescribed medications.
    B. Turning the client every 2 hours.
    C. Instructing the client to use an incentive spirometer twice an hour.
    D. Encouraging the client to drink 2 liters of fluid daily.

2. A 37-year-old client comes into the wellness clinic, stating he has pain. He tells the nurse his antibiotic has given him Red Man syndrome. The nurse is aware which antibiotic is associated with this condition?

    A. Vancomycin
    B. Chloramphenicol
    C. Tetracycline
    D. Erythromycin

3. Which of the following is the priority nursing intervention when an IV infusion infiltrates?

    A. Elevate the site.
    B. Discontinue the infusion.
    C. Apply warm, moist compression.
    D. Contact the healthcare provider.

4. Which of the following ethical principles refers to the duty not to harm?

    A. Veracity
    B. Justice
    C. Non-maleficence
    D. Fidelity

5. A female client in labor is receiving ceftaroline. She suddenly complains of trouble breathing, weakness, and nausea. The nurse should recognize that these signs are usually indicative of impending:

    A. Amniotic fluid embolism
    B. Pulmonary embolism
    C. Anaphylaxis
    D. Bronchospasm

6. Which of the following nursing interventions would be **most** important for determining the fluid balance in a client with end-stage renal failure?

    A. Monitor urine specific gravity.
    B. Measure fluid intake and output.
    C. Monitor daily weights.
    D. Record the frequency of bowel movements.

7. Ms. Johnson presents to the emergency department. Upon assessment, the nurse documents a temperature at 103℉ (39.4℃). She complains of chills, lethargy, and shortness of breath. Infectious endocarditis is suspected. In addition to blood cultures, the nurse would expect Ms. Johnson to undergo which of these diagnostic tests?

    A. Transesophageal echocardiogram
    B. X-ray
    C. B-type natriuretic peptide
    D. Cardiac enzymes

8. A 22-years-old male with a history of sickle cell anemia has an exacerbation of the disease. He states, "I'm getting married and I'm worried about my ability to have sex." Which of these responses by the nurse would be **most** appropriate?

    A. "Is there more you can tell me about it?"
    B. "Have you had any problems with priapism?"
    C. "Have you asked your doctor about sildenafil?"
    D. "What forms of birth control have you been thinking of using?"

9. Which of the following clients is a candidate for treatment with fresh frozen plasma?

    A.   A client with a white blood cell count of 4,000/mm3.
    B.   A client with a platelet count less than 80,000/mm3.
    C.   A preoperative client with an INR of 3.9.
    D.   A postoperative client with a hematocrit of 31%.

10. A nurse is caring for a client 6 hours post right arm mastectomy. Which of the following is correct for client positioning?

    A.   Place the affected arm on a pillow.
    B.   Every 2 hours, turn the client on the prone position on the affected side.
    C.   Place the client in a side-lying position on the unaffected side to promote lymphatic drainage.
    D.   Place the client in semi-Fowler's position.

*How did you do with these management of care questions? How about the priority questions? Take the time to identify what you missed and re-study the content in those specific areas to strengthen your ability to pass NCLEX!*

***Questions can be fun*** *AFTER you've covered your content. If you would like to do more questions just* ***use your phone to scan the code and visit the all new ReMar Nurse Virtual Question Bank!***

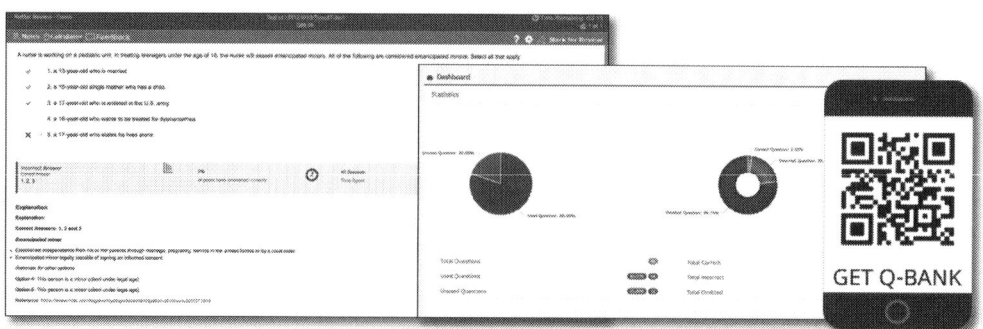

# CLINICAL JUDGEMENT ACTIVITY #18

Circle the client in each group who requires priority assessment.

## Group A

| 1. 33 year old male c/o burnt eyebrows from a fireplace. | 2. A 6 month old male with bulging fontanels crying loudly | 3. A 87 year old female who was found wondering and has not eaten in 3 days. |
|---|---|---|

## Group B

| 1. A four year old girl with a bleeding thumb from a knife trauma | 2. A four year old girl c/o of chest pain with a 02 sat of 99% | 3. A four year old girl with a red swollen wrist from a possible fracture |
|---|---|---|

## Group C

| 1. A 27 year old female with a temperature of 101.0 and diarrhea | 2. A 55 year old male with a kidney stone | 3. A 3 year old female with a cough who is drooling. |
|---|---|---|

## Group D

| 1. A 12 year old with a respiratory infection | 2. A 15 year old with a severed leg and unconscious | 3. A 18 year old c/o chest pain 10/10 |
|---|---|---|

## Group E

| 1. A 10 year old patient with a calcium level of 9.3. | 2. A 20 year old patient with a creatinine level of 2.0. | 3. A 30 year old patient with a BUN level of 18. |
|---|---|---|

## Group F

| 1. A 13 year old female c/o asthma in no respiratory distress | 2. A 22 year old male with a laceration to the chest | 3. A 33 year old c/o body aches, fever, and chills |
|---|---|---|

Group A- Client 1 is the priority as this client has a potential AIRWAY issue due to the burnt eyebrows.

Group B- Client 2 requires additional assessment as chest pain is present without a known cause. The other clients also have circulation issues however their cause is known.

Group C- Client 3 has a possible airway issue as they are drooling which means they are unable to swallow. This may be a suspected sign of epiglottitis.

Group D- Client 2 is unconscious and requires the immediate assessment and intervention to maintain oxygenation.

Group E- Client 2 the normal creatinine level range is 0.5-1.1 mg/dL. This client has an elevated level which indicates the kidney are not functioning properly.

Group F- Client 1 has a breathing issue even though there are no signs of respiratory distress. The condition may be silently getting worse. Immediate assessment is required.

# TIPS TO MASTER NCLEX

| |
|---|
| 1. Content over _____ |
| 2. Forget the real _____ |
| 3. |
| 4. Give yourself permission not to know _____ |
| 5. Confidence is _____. |
| 6. Do not study the day before the exam. |
| 7. You didn't come this far to Fail! |

# TEST DAY TIPS

A. **Know the location (parking, room, etc.)**

B. **Pack everything you need the night before.**

C. **Do not study the night before.**

D. **Eat breakfast and dress in layers.**

E. **Do not go in expecting to stop at minimum questions!**

# NCLEX- RN PRACTICE EXAMS
## FINAL PRACTICE EXAM #1

**Please enter your exam answers in the Virtual Trainer and mark them here in your workbook for your records.**

1. A 42-year-old client is currently abusing heroin and living in a shelter. He states that his current employer is not aware of his living situation. Which response by the nurse is **most** appropriate?

    A. "I must report this information to your current employer to protect the public."
    B. "I must tell your children to protect their safety."
    C. "I will keep everything you tell me confidential."
    D. "I will help you to resolve this issue and explain the matter to all those involved."

2. A 27-year-old male is admitted to the emergency room after a severe motor vehicle accident. The client's Glasgow Coma Scale score is 8. He is showing signs of severe trauma and the doctor would like to place an intracranial pressure catheter. Which of the following is the best method to obtain consent?

    A. Immediately call the client's nearest family member to obtain verbal consent.
    B. The charge nurse is able to sign an emergency consent for the client.
    C. Two physicians will agree that the procedure is necessary and will both sign the consent in an emergency.
    D. The physician will document the emergency and place the catheter without consent. ·

3. A new nurse is preparing to administer blood to a client. The nurse verifies the order and the client's blood type. The nurse should use which of the following to administer the blood?

    A. Nonfiltered tubing with an 18 gauge needle
    B. Micron mesh filter set
    C. Microdrip blood administration set
    D. Clot prevention unfiltered administration set

4. A client who is severely depressed and on suicidal watch tells the nurse, "When I cut myself black tar will spill out of my veins." The nurse knows this is an example of:

    A. Illusion
    B. Hallucination
    C. Delusion
    D. Paranoia

5. A client with a fractured femur has been asked to ambulate without bearing weight on the affected leg. The nurse is satisfied with the client's ambulation if which of the following gaits is demonstrated?

    A. Two-point gait
    B. Four-point gait
    C. Swing to gait
    D. Three-point gait

6. A nurse is working on a long term care unit and is caring for a client on parenteral nutrition. The nurse notices the supplement feeding bag is running low. What fluid should she have on hand?

    A. 10% Dextrose
    B. 0.9% Normal saline
    C. 2% Glucose in amino acids
    D. 45% Glucose in water

7. The nurse is assisting a client using topical Gentamicin sulfate. Which of the following comments by the clients need follow-up teaching?

    A. I will continue to apply this medication ten days after the infection clears up.
    B. I will contact my physician if the condition worsens.
    C. I will avoid being out in the sun for long periods.
    D. I can cover the infected area with gauze dressing if I desire.

8. A client has been taking imipramine for his depression for 4 days. His wife asks the nurse, "Why is he still so depressed?" Which of the following responses by the nurse is most appropriate?

    A. Let's look over this chart to see if there are possible drug interactions.
    B. It takes 2-4 weeks for the drug to reach its full effect.
    C. The severity of the depression will determine how soon the medication works.
    D. I will have the physician speak with you concerning this medication.

9. A nurse is caring for a client on an acute psychiatric unit. Which interventions should the nurse use to assist the client with mood-congruent delusions?

    A. Confronting the client's delusions
    B. Engaging the client only when he is engaged in reality
    C. Accepting the client while not arguing with the delusion
    D. Focusing on the definition of a delusion.

10. The nurse coordinates with the laboratory staff to have the gentamicin trough serum level drawn. At what time should the blood be drawn in relation to the administration of the next IV dose of gentamicin?

    A. 2 hours before the administration of the next IV dose.
    B. 3 hours before the administration of the next IV dose.
    C. 1 hour before the administration of the next IV dose.
    D. Just before the administration of the next IV dose.

11. A 3-year-old is admitted to the emergency room with a sudden temperature of 102. F, sore throat, and drooling saliva. The child is leaning forward and will not lie down supine for an exam. Which of the following should the nurse do next?

    A. Give 500 mg of acetaminophen rectally.
    B. Obtain a sputum specimen to culture any bacteria
    C. Gather an appropriate sized tracheostomy kit.
    D. Assess the child's throat while they are sitting on the parent's lap.

12. A client is on levothyroxine and asks the nurse how long she has to take this medication for hypothyroidism. The nurse should respond by saying.

    A. This medication will be taken daily for the rest of your life.
    B. The medication dose can be reduced if you are worried about the expenses.
    C. The medication will be tapered off after 2 to 3 years of controlled usage.
    D. The medication can be tapered off once the thyroid-stimulating hormone returns to normal.

13. A client with an intestinal bleed is vomiting bright red blood. His hemoglobin level is 6 g/DL, and his blood pressure is 90/45. The client and his family are Jehovah's Witness and do not believe in administering blood or blood products. The nurse should prepare to do which of the following interventions.

    A. Disregard a consent due to an emergency and administer frozen plasma.
    B. Educate the family on the difference between frozen plasma and packed red blood cells.
    C. Attempt to stabilize the client with IV fluids.
    D. Notify the hospital ethics committee to protect the client.

14. A client with a history of myocardial infarction carries nitroglycerin on them at all times. The nurse instructs the client that the nitroglycerin should be kept in:

    A. In a refrigerator, if the nitroglycerin is transdermal.
    B. In a dark container shielded from light.
    C. A cool moist place.
    D. In a pocket instead of a handbag which may difficult to reach.

15. A client is recuperating after a myocardial infarction and wants to increase his activity. The nurse should monitor the client for which of the following conditions while he engages in increased activity?

    A. Dyspnea
    B. Weight gain
    C. Edema
    D. Crackles

16. The nurse is preparing a client who is newly diagnosed with Biermer's disease. Which is the first step in the teaching process?

    A. Choose the best reading materials.
    B. Determine the learning needs of the client.
    C. Set the priorities of the learning needs.
    D. Determine the goals of the teaching environment.

17. Which of the following is an adverse effect of clindamycin and needs to be reported to the physician immediately?

    A. Tinnitus
    B. Ataxia
    C. Abdominal Pain
    D. Yellow halos

18. A client has just returned from a bronchoscopy and an emergency biopsy. The nurse is aware which of the following signs should be reported immediately to the physician?

    A. Frequent dry cough
    B. Blood streaked sputum
    C. Laryngeal stridor
    D. Green sputum

19. A nurse is reporting for duty. She has just received a report on four clients. Which should she see first?

    A. The client who has been deceased for 1 hour.
    B. A client who reports he may have splashed a harmful chemical in his eyes
    C. A client reporting abdominal pain from a kidney stone
    D. A client who is reporting pain from a splint that was placed too tightly.

20. A nurse has signed on for duty. She has just received report on four clients. Which should she see first?

    A. A client admitted with tuberculosis and a fever of 102.4
    B. A client reporting of SOB when eating.
    C. A client reporting abdominal pain 7 hours after a PEG tube placement.
    D. A client with a decreased pedal pulse diagnosed with peripheral artery disease.

21. A nurse is reporting for duty. She has just received an assignment of four clients. Which should she see first?

    A. A client on a nitroglycerin drip
    B. A client on a morphine drip
    C. A client on a potassium drip
    D. A client on a magnesium drip

22. Which is the priority nursing intervention for a client who is brought to the emergency room with burns over approximately 45% of the body surface area?

    A. Insert a patent IV line to administer isotonic fluids
    B. Administer morphine to decrease pain and prevent shock
    C. Establish an airway
    D. Assess burn density to determine whether it is chemical or electrical before administering any treatment.

23. A 47-year-old client is admitted to the intensive care unit with complications from a stroke 10 hours ago. A dislodged clot caused the stroke. The nurse anticipates seeing which of the following on the client's electrocardiogram strip?

    A. Ventricular tachycardia
    B. Normal sinus rhythm
    C. Atrial fibrillation
    D. Ventricular fibrillation

24. A nurse has just received a client who is 2 hours post hernia repair from the post-anesthesia care unit PACU. Upon doing the primary survey, she notices the abdominal incision eviscerates. The nurse should do which of the following first?

    A. Begin a bolus of normal saline
    B. Cover the incision with a dressing moistened with normal saline
    C. Put the client in the reverse Trendelenburg position
    D. Assess the client's pain and call the physician

25. A client has just lost an arm from a motor vehicle accident. The client was medicated for pain and tells the nurse. "I was so scared from the pain; I didn't think I was going to make it." Which is the best response by the nurse?

    A. You always have medication available do not be afraid of pain.
    B. Why did you think you were going to die?
    C. I understand that pain can be a frightening experience.
    D. Please take the medication before you upset yourself more.

26. A client with cholecystitis is taking propantheline bromide. The expected effect of this drug is:

    A. Increased bile production
    B. Decreased biliary spasm
    C. Decrease infections
    D. Improved urine output

27. A nurse is aware of the use of restraints. She knows which of the following statements are false.

    A. Restraints can be a part of PRN orders
    B. The use of restraints should be a part of a comprehensive assessment.
    C. The use of restraints should not be considered based on a client's past violent behavior.
    D. Reorientation is an acceptable practice to delay the use of restraints.

28. A nurse is aware of the use of restraints. Chose the statement that should be refuted.

    A. A registered nurse can initiate a restraint if alternatives are not successful.
    B. A physician's order is not required for a restraint.
    C. A restraint order needs to be renewed every 12 hours.
    D. The type of restraint must be clearly documented in the order.
    E. Clients in restraints need to have care documented every 2 hours.

29. A licensed practical nurse (LPN) is reporting to the emergency department for a floating assignment. The charge nurse knows which client is most appropriate to give the LPN.

    A. A client who is waiting to be admitted for unrelieved chest pain.
    B. A client who was admitted 6 hours ago with hemophilia
    C. A client with burns to the face and neck
    D. A client awaiting surgery for a brain aneurysm.

30. Immediately after a percutaneous liver biopsy, the nurse should place the client in which of the following positions?

    A. Supine.
    B. Right side-lying.
    C. Left side-lying.
    D. Semi-Fowler's.

31. A nurse has checked the residuals on her client with a g-tube. The client has severe, delayed gastric emptying and a decreased level of consciousness. Which position is most beneficial to this client?

    A. Right side-lying with the head of bed elevated
    B. Left side-lying with the head of bed elevated
    C. Low fowler's position
    D. Trendelenburg

32. An infant with spina bifida is being hospitalized. The mother wants to feed the child. Which position is most appropriate?

    A. Supine
    B. Semi-fowlers
    C. Prone
    D. Lying flat with legs elevated

33. The nurse believes a coworker is diverting narcotics. The nurse approaches the nurse manager to report the suspicions. Which of the following statements by the nurse is best?

    A. After my coworker ends a shift, the clients need repeated doses of pain medication. I have also witnessed her sleeping on the job four times.
    B. I saw my coworker downtown after work. She was acting strange like she didn't even recognize me.
    C. I believe my coworker is stealing narcotics because she is always looking high.
    D. I saw what I believe to be tracks on my coworker's arms, and I think she hangs out in a drug house.

34. The nurse plans care for a 36-year-old woman with Graves' disease. The nurse knows that which of the following foods or fluids should be restricted for this client?

    A. Ice cream
    B. Tea
    C. Oranges
    D. Pasta

35. A client had a thoracotomy 4 hours ago. For the past 2 hours, there has been 100 ml per hour of bloody chest drainage. Which of the following actions should the nurse take first?

    A. Assess the chest tube set-up
    B. Assess the dressing for excessive blood
    C. Call the physician
    D. Elevate the head of the bed

36. A nurse is caring for a client newly diagnosed with chronic obstructive pulmonary disorder. Which activity is the best for this client?

    A. isometric leg exercise
    B. lumbar-sacral exercise
    C. pursed-lip breathing
    D. intercostal muscle expansion

37. Which action should the nurse take first when she observes a client with an untreated right pneumothorax?

    A. Assist the client in coughing and deep breathing
    B. Administer sedative
    C. Prepare to insert chest drainage system
    D. Prepare the client for CT

38. A nurse is starting her shift. She is given report on four clients. Which should she see first?

    A. A client who recently started tube feeding and has three loose stools in the last 5 hours
    B. A client who has a newly inserted bladder catheter and is apprehensive and complaining of itching
    C. A client who recently had a thoracotomy and complaining of pain at the insertion site
    D. A client who newly was diagnosed with systemic lupus erythematosus complaining of redness of the palms

39. A client on a ventilator is diagnosed with stage 4 lung cancer. The nurse enters the room, and the client's high-pressure alarm is sounding. The nurse knows the cause of this alarm is which of the following?

    A. The client needs to be suctioned
    B. The client has become disconnected from the ventilator
    C. There is a crack in the ventilator tubing allowing air to seep out
    D. There is a leak around the ET tube

40. A nurse is entering a client's room after doing her morning rounds. The client's ventilator alarm is sounding and the nurse is unable to identify the issue. Which is the initial action of the nurse?

    A. Call respiratory therapy for help
    B. Disconnect the client from the and use a manual resuscitation bag
    C. Place the client in high fowler's position immediately
    D. Disconnect the client and begin CPR

# REMAR REVIEW SELECT ALL THAT APPLY PRACTICE EXAM

Please enter your exam answers in the Virtual Trainer and mark them here in your workbook for your records.

1. A new nurse is working in the emergency department. He is aware he must report the following?
   Select all that apply.

   A. A child bitten by a dog
   B. A child who states he doesn't eat lunch
   C. A child has bruises on his left earlobe
   D. A child who accidentally ingested some toilet bowl cleaner
   E. A child who has drawn a sexually inappropriate picture

2. While a nurse is performing CPR she should do which of the following? Select all that apply.

   A. Ensure full chest recoil
   B. Rotate compressions every 1 minute with rhythm checks
   C. Give 2 breaths per 5 cycles that are less than 3 minutes
   D. Initiate hyperventilation
   E. Push hard and fast

3. A nurse is preparing to care for a client diagnosed with a recent cerebral vascular accident. The client is diagnosed with a hemorrhagic stroke. The nurse should expect which of the following medications to be administered? Select all that apply.

   A. Nitroprusside
   B. Labetalol
   C. Fibrinolytic treatment
   D. Aspirin
   E. Glucagon

4. Which of the following is true concerning Judaism? Select all that apply.

   A. Meats allowed include animals that have uncloven hoofs
   B. Only 1 combination of meat and milk is acceptable
   C. Yom Kippur is a ritual time of fasting
   D. Fish that have scales and fins are allowed
   E. During Passover week, only leavened bread is allowed

5. A nurse is caring for a client prescribed lindane for head lice. Which of the following statements require follow-up teaching? Select all that apply.

   A. "All members of my household should be treated."
   B. "This medication is safe for my wife who is breastfeeding."
   C. "This medication should not be used for children under 2."
   D. "This medication may cause alopecia."
   E. "Lindane may increase blood glucose levels in patients with diabetes mellitus."

6. A nurse is aware which of the following is true regarding testicular cancer? Select all that apply.

   A. Testicular cancer is the least common solid tumor in young males
   B. There is usually a non-tender irregular mass
   C. Seminomas make up 90% of testicular cancer
   D. Self-examination is important to identify future tumors
   E. Chemotherapy is not effective with testicular cancer

7. A nurse is caring for a 66 years old male client who is newly prescribed a vasodilator. Which of the following is a concern when using vasodilatory medication in the elderly? Select all that apply

    A. Pedal edema
    B. Renal failure
    C. Headaches
    D. Orthostatic hypotension
    E. Vitamin B-13 deficiency

8. A nurse is caring for a client who just received a 12 lead EKG. The rhythm showed Mobitz type II second degree heart block. Which of the following will be a part of the treatment plan? Select all that apply.

    A. Atropine 0.5 mg IV while waiting for pacing
    B. Atropine 0.5 mg IV while awaiting cardioversion
    C. Transcutaneous pacing
    D. Cardioversion
    E. Defibrillation
    F. Fibrinolytics

9. Which of the following is considered a part of the continuity of care responsibilities for a staff nurse? Select all that apply.

    A. Handoff reporting
    B. Discharge planning
    C. Transfer reporting
    D. Coordinating community resources
    E. Verifying insurance claims

10. A nurse is caring for a client diagnosed with end-stage renal disease with current blood pressure 70/40, a heart rate of 105, and respirations 23. Which of the following nursing interventions should the nurse expect to administer? Select all that apply.

    A. Administer Nitroprusside IV to restore blood volume
    B. Notify the laboratory to draw a hemoglobin level
    C. Initiate an IV and administer 0.9 normal saline
    D. Initiate an IV and administer Methotrexate
    E. Apply supplemental oxygen

11. A nurse is aware which of the following is true about conducting a physical assessment? Select all that apply.

    A. It is done best when comparing the right and left side of the body
    B. It is done in the order of inspection, palpation, percussion, auscultation
    C. Vibration is the best palpated using the ulnar surface of the hand
    D. It is best conducted by standing on the foot of the examination table
    E. It should be conducted in a toe to head approach

12. A nurse is caring for a client with a T3 spinal cord injury. The client complains of nausea, sweating, and feeling dizzy. The client is hypertensive and anxious. Which of the following nursing interventions is most appropriate? Select all that apply.

    A. Inquire about the client's feeling of anxiety
    B. Start the client on a 0.9 normal saline bolus
    C. Assess the client for bladder distention
    D. Sit the client in high fowler's position
    E. Administer prescribed anti-hypertensive

13. A nurse is caring for a child diagnosed with Attention Deficit Hyperactivity Disorder. Which of the following medications could the client be prescribed? Select all that apply.

    A. Amphetamine
    B. Dextroamphetamine
    C. Pemoline
    D. Methylphenidate
    E. Methamphetamine

14. Which of the following actions that nurses are legally responsible for? Select all that apply.

    A. Safely handling and storing medication
    B. Determining if a medication order was written correctly
    C. Reporting all medication errors
    D. Inform the client if the physician is not qualified to treat their condition
    E. Having knowledge of federal policies that regulate the safe prescribing of medication

15. A nurse is preparing to administer a medication that blocks sympathetic nervous system stimulation of the heart rate and sympathetic vasoconstriction. The client was diagnosed with primary hypertension. Which of the following is a contraindication to administering this medication? Select all that apply.

    A. Heart rate <60 bpm
    B. PR interval >0.24 seconds
    C. Acute asthma
    D. History of deep vein thrombosis
    E. Current use of Enoxaparin 30 mg IV

16. A new nurse is orientating on the newborn nursery unit. The nurse is aware which of the following should be included in the Apgar score assessment? Select all that apply.

    A. Heart Rate
    B. Temperature
    C. Respirations
    D. Muscle tone
    E. Color
    F. Blood pressure
    G. Reflexes

17. The physician prescribed naloxone to be given to reverse the effects of a narcotic overdose. The nurse is aware the medication can be given which routes? Select all that apply.

    A. SL
    B. IV
    C. Nasal spray
    D. IM
    E. SQ

18. A nurse is caring for a client who has multiple mouth ulcers. The client is placed on a clear liquid diet. Select all the items that are allowed on the dietary tray.

    A. Hospital issued vegetable juice
    B. Gelatin
    C. Broth
    D. Pudding
    E. Pureed vegetables
    F. Coffee
    G. Chicken soup

19. A new nurse is aware the risks of central line placement. Which of the following are potential risks of central line placement? Select all that apply.

    A. Fatigue
    B. Air embolism
    C. Fluid overload
    D. Infection
    E. Hyperglycemia
    F. Hypomagnesemia
    G. Dehydration .

20. Which of the following is true about the effects of a lumbar epidural block? Select all that apply.

    A. The anesthesia should be administered after labor is established
    B. The anesthetic numbs the vagina
    C. The anesthetic may cause maternal hypotension
    D. The injection site is in the epidural space at L3-L4
    E. The anesthetic relieves pain from contractions

21. What information should the nurse include when teaching post circumcision care to parents of a newborn before discharge from the hospital? Select all that apply:

    A. The infant must void before being discharged home
    B. Petroleum jelly should be applied to the glans of the penis with each diaper change
    C. The infant can take tub baths while the circumcision heals
    D. Any blood noted on the front of the diaper should be reported
    E. The circumcision will require care for 2 to 4 days after discharge

22. A nurse working in a psychiatric unit is helping to admit a suicidal client. How should the nurse respond when the client asks, "How long do I have to stay here?" Select all that apply.

    A. You should stay until you are safe but we can discuss this more after you are assessed by the whole health team
    B. You will be here until you are free from harm
    C. A lawyer will help you to determine when is the best time to leave
    D. Once you sign your treatment admission papers, you are committed to the psychiatric safety unit
    E. The attending physician will let you know the length of stay he is prescribing.

23. A client is admitted to the outpatient surgery center for a liver biopsy. Which of the following laboratory tests assesses coagulation? Select all that apply.

    A. Partial thromboplastin time
    B. Complete blood count
    C. Platelet count
    D. Hemoglobin
    E. Hematocrit
    F. White blood cell count

24. The nurse is teaching the client how to use a metered-dose inhaler (MDI) to administer a corticosteroid drug. Which of the following client actions indicates that he is using the MDI correctly? Select all that apply.

    A. The client lies supine for 15 minutes following administration
    B. The client waits 5 minutes between each puff
    C. The inhaler is tilted while inhaling the medication
    D. The client rinses his mouth after taking medication
    E. The inhaler is held upright while taking medication

25. A nurse is caring for a client with ulcerative colitis who is experiencing symptoms, which client care activities can the nurse appropriately delegate to an unlicensed assistant? Select all that apply.

   A. Assisting the client with taking his oral antacid reflux drink
   B. Providing skincare after a bowel movement
   C. Assessing the client's response to ambulation therapy
   D. Maintaining accurate intake records
   E. Obtaining the client's weight

26. Which of the following nursing instructions are written incorrectly? Select all that apply.

   A. Change dressing every shift
   B. Elevate the head of bed 45 degrees after meals
   C. Apply heating pad during day
   D. Perform neuro checks
   E. Ambulate down the hall 6 feet BID

27. The nurse is monitoring a client receiving peritoneal dialysis, and nurse notes that a client's outflow is less than the inflow. Which actions should the nurse take? Select all that apply.

   A. Place the client in proper body alignment
   B. Check the level of the drainage bag
   C. Contact the physician
   D. Check the peritoneal dialysis system for kinks
   E. Reposition the client to his or her side

The answers to your **Select All That Apply Exam** are provided on the following pages.

The recommended score is 25 out of 27 correct

# REMAR REVIEW SELECT ALL THAT APPLY PRACTICE EXAM ANSWERS

1. All of the situations must be reported by nurses
A. A child not eating a meal is a form of neglect, the child was not protected from harm
B. The child is not receiving adequate nutrition. This is a form of abuse and should be reported.
C. This child has a sign of physical abuse, and it needs to should be reported.
D. This is a form of neglect, and the child was not protected from a dangerous poison.
E. This is a sign of potential sexual abuse

2. A, E are correct. The nurse should ensure full chest recoil when administering chest compressions. The nurse should also push down hard and fast at a rate of 100 compressions per minute for all victims except newborns. Item B is incorrect as compressions should be rotated every 2 minutes with rhythm checks. C is incorrect. It is recommended to give two breaths per 5 cycles that are less than 2 minutes D is also incorrect the nurse should avoid hyperventilation.

3. A, B are correct. A cerebral vascular stroke can be caused by bleeding so the client should avoid all blood thinners such as coumadin and aspirin. The client's condition would also be contraindicated for fibrinolytic therapy. Glucagon is not initially indicated.

4. C, D are correct statements following Judaism. A is an incorrect choice as the meats allowed include animals with cloven hoofs B. No combination of milk and meat is acceptable. E was also incorrect as during Passover week, only unleavened bread is allowed

5. A and C are correct. B is incorrect as the medication lindane is not safe for a woman who are breastfeeding. D. 'This medication may cause alopecia- is not true." "Lindane may increase blood glucose levels in patients with diabetes mellitus this is not true."

6. B, C, D are correct item options. A is incorrect as testicular cancer is the most common solid tumor in young males. Item E is incorrect because chemotherapy and radiation are effective treatment methods.

7. C and D are correct. The medication is a vasodilator which one would expect a side effect to be orthostatic hypotension and headaches. The other items are non-related.

8. A and C are correct. Atropine and transcutaneous pacing are viable treatment options for second-degree heart block. All of the other options are not a current treatment option for Mobitz Type II second degree heart block.

9. A, B, and C are part of the staff nurse duties. D and E, which are coordinating community resources, are part of case management duties.

10. C, E are correct. Item A to give nitroprusside is inappropriate as it would further decrease the blood pressure. Item B is not necessary and does not help restore blood volume. Item D methotrexate is a medication used for cancer, not hypotension.

11. A, B, & C are correct. D is incorrect as the examiner should start at the head of the bed and move down according to the exam. E is wrong as the physical assessment should be done in a head to toe approach.

12. C, D, & E are correct as the client is experiencing signs of possible autonomic dysreflexia. The nurse should assess the client for bladder distention, place the client in a high fowler's position. It is also appropriate to administer prescribed antihypertensive medication. Item A is not addressing the autonomic dysreflexia that is occurring. B is not an appropriate intervention as intravenous fluids could further increase blood pressure.

13. A, B, C, D, & E are all correct. Stimulant medications including amphetamines such as dextroamphetamine, methamphetamine, methylphenidate are considered effective treatments for attention hyperactivity disorder. Pemoline is a central nervous system depressant that is also effective for the treatment of ADHD.

14. A, B, C, & E are all correct actions that a nurse is legally responsible to do. Item D of knowing if a physician meets practice qualifications is not the legal responsibility of the nurse. This not the duty of the nurse but of the physician to be truthful about their skills.

15. A, B, and C are correct. The medication described is a beta-blocker. The nurse should not administer if the client's HR is less than 60. If the cardiac PR interval is increased, it indicates a heart block is present. The beta-blocker medication would further increase the abnormal PR interval. This could negatively affect tissue perfusion. Clients with respiratory issues such as acute asthma should not take beta-blockers, which could produce respiratory distress or produce asthmatic attacks. Items D and E are unrelated to the administration of beta-blockers.

16. A, C, D, E, & G are the correct item choices. Heart rate, respiration, muscle tone, color, and reflexes are assessment markers when calculating an APGAR score. All the other item choices are not included in the Apgar score.

17. A, B, D & E are the correct item choices. Naloxone can be given the sublingual, intravenous, intramuscular, and subcutaneous route. Naloxone is not a nasal spray.

18. B, C, F are correct item choices. A clear liquid diet helps maintain adequate hydration, provides important electrolytes. Gelatin, broth, and coffee are acceptable items on the clear liquid diet.

19. B, C, and D are correct item choices. A central venous catheter, also known as a central line, is a tube that doctors place in a large vein in the neck, chest, groin, or arm to give fluids, blood, or medications or to do medical tests quickly. A venous air embolism occurs when air enters the venous system and eventually causes an obstruction in the pulmonary circulation. Air emboli exist only when there is a connection between the air and the vascular system. Central lines are commonly used for rapid fluid resuscitation. Complications of fluid overload must be evaluated when a central line is placed. Infection is a serious complication of a central line insertion.
Fatigue, hyperglycemia, hypomagnesemia, and dehydration are not directly associated with central line placement.

20. A, B, C, D, & E are correct item choices. Anesthesia should not be administered before true labor has been established as it could stall progression. The anesthetic will numb the vaginal area. The purpose of the epidural is to provide pain relief during uterine contractions. The most common complications occurring with epidural analgesia are maternal hypotension and post-dural puncture headache. The injection site of the needle is between the lamina of the vertebrae L3-L4.

21.A, B, & E are all correct. Circumcision is the surgical removal of the foreskin that covers the head of the penis. It is an elective procedure based on the parents' choice. The infant must void urine before discharge is appropriate. Petroleum jelly should be applied to the glans of the penis to avoid the discomfort of sticking to the diaper. It will take approximately two to four days to heal. The parents should avoid tub baths until the circumcision heals. Small amounts of blood should not be reported as they are a normal part of the healing process.

22. A and B are correct item choices. The nurse should provide reassurance to the client. The nurse has the responsibility of informing the client of the possible treatment plan. The goal of the treatment is to prevent the client from harming themselves or others. Items C, D, and E are in =correct. A lawyer will not determine the length of time a client requires treatment. Unless a court order is involved, the client will not be required to receive treatment.

23. A & C are the correct choices. Partial thromboplastin time and platelet count are all included in coagulation studies. The hemoglobin, hematocrit, and white blood count are important laboratory values but does not assess coagulation.

24. B, D, & E are correct item options. A metered-dose inhaler, called an MDI for short, is a pressurized inhaler that delivers medication by using a propellant spray. The client should wait 3 to 5 minutes between each puff. Mouth washing after inhalation of corticosteroids is effective for prevention of local adverse effects such as hoarseness and oropharyngeal candidiasis. The inhaler should be held upright for medication to be properly administered.

25. B, D, & E are correct item options. The unlicensed assistive personnel should be given activities that support daily living such as feeding and dressing.
The UAP should not give medication to clients. The UAP is not able to assess responses to therapy.

26. A, C, are D are the correct item choices. These orders are written incorrectly. The order to change the dressing every shift does not give a type of dressing to perform. The order to apply a heating pad during the day does not give a location, time limit, or frequency. The order to perform neurological checks does not give a frequency. The other item choices are written correctly.

27. A, B, D, E are correct item options. If the outflow is inadequate, the nurse attempts to stimulate outflow by changing the client's position. Turning the client to the other side or making sure that the client is in proper body alignment may assist with outflow drainage. The drainage bag needs to be lower than the client's abdomen to enhance gravity drainage. The connecting tubing and the peritoneal dialysis system is also checked for kinks or twisting, and the clamps on the system are tested to ensure that they are open. At the specific moment, there is no reason to contact the physician.

1.) A client's physician has placed him on a low sodium diet; select the following food that should be avoided because it is high in sodium:

   A.   Milk
   B.   Frozen vegetables
   C.   Butter
   D.   Orange Juice
   E.   Peaches

2.) A nurse is taking care of an elderly client with significant tremors. Which of these assistive devices would be most beneficial to this client for his activities of daily living?

   A.   Arm lifter
   B.   Voice amplifier
   C.   Buttonhook
   D.   Flashlight

3.) Cimetidine should not be taken with the following medication:

   A.   Potassium
   B.   Coumadin
   C.   Grape Juice
   D.   Epinephrine

4.) Peptic ulcer disease is associated with smoking and stress. The treatment can be multifocal and intensive. Select the treatment option that is associated with peptic ulcer disease:

   A.   Treat the bacteria Helicobacter pylori
   B.   Teaching the client to chew proton pump inhibitors with meals
   C.   Teach the client to take over the counter hydrocortisone
   D.   Teach the client to avoid antacids

5.) A mother brings her child into the emergency room and the baby is pronounced dead due to sudden infant death syndrome (SIDS). Which question is appropriate for the nurse to ask the parents?

   A.   Did you have any education on the risk factors associated with sudden infant death syndrome?
   B.   Can you explain possible reasons why this happened to your child?
   C.   Are there siblings at home that need to be cared for?
   D.   This could have happened when you placed toys in the crib.

6.) A nurse is providing education to new parents regarding sudden infant death syndrome (SIDS). The nurse should include these statements during the instruction: Select all that apply.

   A    SIDS can occur in healthy babies
   B.   The cause of SIDS is an abnormal respiratory pattern
   C.   A brown eyes is a risk factor
   D.   Make sure to put all babies to sleep in a prone position
   E.   Only one stuffed animal is allowed in the crib with the infant

7.) A client has a new stoma from an ileal conduit. Which statement by the client verbalizes understanding of the skincare?

    A.   I can no longer participate in contact sports
    B.   I should change my stoma appliance during the early morning
    C.   I can leave my stoma open to air when I go swimming
    D.   I should wash the area around my stoma with antimicrobial soap to prevent infection

8.) When caring for a client with an indwelling urinary catheter the nurse knows to do which of the following:

    A.   Lay the urinary collection bag on the floor to promote drainage
    B.   Insert the urinary catheter carefully using a clean technique
    C.   Do frequent assessments to make sure the drainage system is closed at all times
    D.   Clean the meatus with 10% betadine daily to prevent infection

9.) The nurse is preparing to administer zolpidem tartrate 5mg PO to a client before bedtime. The nurse should make which of the following statements concerning sleep therapy with zolpidem tartrate?

    A.   Take this only when you can sleep for at least 8 hours
    B.   Take this medication on an empty stomach before dinner
    C.   This medication is for the long term treatment of insomnia
    D.   This medication will allow you to operate heavy machinery safely

10.) A client is admitted to the cardiology unit with a diagnosis of congestive heart failure. Upon auscultation of the lungs, the nurse notices a snapping sound caused by the alveoli being opened on inspiration and expiration. This is which of the following?

    A.   Crepitus
    B.   Tactile fremitus
    C.   Crackles
    D.   Egophony

11.) What physical finding would be expected during the initial assessment of a client with long term emphysema?

    A.   Increased jugular distention
    B.   Clubbing of the fingers
    C.   Varicose veins
    D.   Paronychia

12.) A high pitched musical sound heard during auscultation is referred to as:

    A.   Tactile fremitus
    B.   Wheeze
    C.   Rhonchi
    D.   Rales

13.) A client comes to the emergency room and is diagnosed with scarlet fever. Scarlet fever may follow which type of infection?

    A.   Urinary tract infection
    B.   Intestinal infection
    C.   Strep throat infection
    D.   Pinworm infection

14.) As the nurse of the client with scarlet fever, you know to initiate which type of isolation precaution?

    A.   Airborne
    B.   Contact
    C.   Droplet
    D.   Standard

15.) Clients with HIV are given highly active antiretroviral therapy (HAART) to treat infections and prevent complications. The client will be at risk for opportunistic infections when his CD4 count is below:

    A.   200
    B.   300
    C.   400
    D.   500

16.) A pregnant client is admitted to the hospital and diagnosed with pre-eclampsia; she is at risk for premature labor. The healthcare provider orders magnesium sulfate 5 grams IV. The nurse is aware the client will need which intervention after the medication is given?

    A.   Placement of an indwelling catheter
    B.   A heating pad to prevent hypothermia
    C.   Calcium decanoate at the bedside for possible toxicity
    D.   An arterial blood gas reading within 2 hours due to potential respiratory depression

17.) After an unsuccessful sky dive, a client's Glasgow Coma Scale score is 6. The nurse would expect this client's level of consciousness to be which of the following?

    A.   Alert but confused
    B.   Drowsy
    C.   Stuporus
    D.   Comatose

18.) Place the methods of a physical examination on the abdomen in order. Select the correct options and then sequence the items in the correct order.

    A. Percussion
    B. Palpitation
    C. Auscultation
    D. Visualization
    E. Inspection
    F. Manipulation

---

19.) A client is requesting food after a bronchoscopy. The nurse obtains a positive gag reflex. A positive gag reflex means which cranial nerve is intact?

    A.   CN III
    B.   CNIV
    C.   CN VII
    D.   CN X

20.) A mother brings her 18-month-old child to the clinic for a routine assessment and vaccinations. Which task would the nurse expect the child to have mastered?

    A.   The ability to walk
    B.   The ability to say 12 words
    C.   The child is toilet trained
    A.   The child can count to 3

Mark your answers in the book and enter the answer into your virtual trainer. The answers will be there. After each question mark whether you got it correct or not. You must get a 95% on this exam! If you don't hit the 95% go back and study the content areas of your incorrect answers. Get them wrong here and right on NCLEX!

# NCLEX-RN FINAL PRACTICE EXAM QUESTIONS 3

Please enter your exam answers in the Virtual Trainer and mark them here in your workbook for your records.

1. A client is diagnosed with systemic lupus erythematosus. Which of the following is a classic sign?

   A. Skin lesions on the face
   B. Bronchospasms
   C. Blood clots
   D. Difficulty swallowing

2. A client who had a left above the knee amputation one day ago was transferred to the rehabilitation center. Upon admission, the nurse notices the client's compression bandage has slipped off, which action should the nurse take **first**?

   A. Place the client in the left side-lying position
   B. Elevate the left leg on 1-2 pillows and write a note
   C. Notify the on-call physician
   D. Replace the compression bandage

3. The charge nurse must notify a staff member to stay home because of low census. The unit currently has 35 clients whom all have at least one IV and multiple oral medications. The unit is staffed with two RNs, three licensed practical nurses (LPNs), and three unlicensed assistive personnel (UAPs).
   Which nurse should be notified to stay home?

   1. The least experienced RN.
   2. The most experienced LPN.
   3. The UAP who asked to be requested off.
   4. The UAP who was hired 4 weeks ago.

4. A nurse is caring for a client who is a recent amputee. She understands which nursing intervention is **best** for the prevention of external rotation of the affected limb?

   A. Putting a pillow under the leg while in the supine position
   B. Applying a sandbag to the knee of the affected leg
   C. Covering the skin breakdown with a prosthesis to keep infection away
   D. Dusting the affected limb with talcum powder before applying the prosthesis

5. Which of the following activities should the nurse plan to teach the client to strengthen his hand muscles in preparation for using crutches?

   A. Eating her meals with a spoon
   B. Incorporating push-ups into the exercise routine
   C. Squeezing a softball
   D. Combing her hair independently

6. A nurse is preparing to testify in court about a client who was admitted to the medical unit. The client fell out of bed after having a seizure. On admission, the nurse initiated seizure precautions. After the nurse's shift, the client fell out of bed. During the court hearing, which of the following should the nurse be prepared to testify about?

   A. The client's mental status during the fall.
   B. How the client fell out of the bed.
   C. The facility's seizure precaution protocol.
   D. The client's injuries after the fall out of bed.

7. A client recently placed in a nursing home states to the nurse, "My family doesn't love me. They want me to hurry up and die." Which of the following is the **best** response by the nurse?

    A. Were you causing trouble for them at home?
    B. Why do you feel so depressed?
    C. Can I call your family and speak to them?
    D. Can you tell me more about your feelings?

8. A 60-year-old client is admitted for a surgical repair of an abdominal aortic aneurysm. The history includes diabetes for 15 years, hyperlipidemia for nine years, and smoking for 50 years. The client asks the nurse what caused the aneurysm. The nurse's **best** response should be:

    A. Lack of exercise caused the aneurysm
    B. Plague which leads to atherosclerosis may lead to aneurysms
    C. Infections from diabetes can lead to aneurysms
    D. A congenital defect is most likely the cause of your aneurysm

9. A nurse working in a nursing home observes four new bruises on a female resident's arms and back. Which intervention should the nurse implement **first**?

    A. Check the client's medication record to see if an anticoagulant medication was given
    B. File an elder abuse report
    C. Notify the client's family of the bruises before they arrive
    D. Ask the client about the bruises
    E. Notify the healthcare provider

10. The nurse is preparing to administer 250,000 units of medication to a client. The ampule sent from the pharmacy contains 500,000 units/mL. How many mL should the nurse administer?

    A. 0.5 ml
    B. 1.0 ml
    C. 250,000 ml
    D. 50,000 ml

11. The nurse is caring for a teenage client diagnosed with syphilis. Besides administering the medication, what other actions should the nurse anticipate in the **initial** treatment?

    A. Suggesting the client also take a multi-vitamin supplement
    B. Instructing the client about the risk of other sexually transmitted diseases
    C. Identifying all sexual partners
    D. Educating the client on the complications of not thoroughly treating the infection.

12. A 28-year-old female is seen in the gynecologic client. The nurse should plan to begin her interview with which of the following?

    A. Sexual history including the number of partners in the last year
    B. Urinary system history to include treatment for venereal diseases
    C. Obstetric history to include the number of pregnancies, live births and any abortions
    D. Menstrual history to include any issues such as irregular periods

13. The **most** appropriate nursing intervention to encourage a non-verbal, depressed client would be to:

    A. discuss threatening subjects
    B. ask the client to share openly
    C. ask very simple questions that require simple answers
    D. sit with the client for short periods of time

14. The nurse is caring for a client who is hallucinating. The client tells the nurse "I didn't kill the man, you know I didn't do it. Please tell them the truth!" The nurse should respond by saying:

    A. Who did you kill?
    B. Do not become too upset; we are in this together.
    C. No one is talking to you; this is part of your illness.
    D. I realize you must be very scared.

15. A retired military veteran frequently visits the community health center with multiple vague complaints of abdominal pain. Although no physical cause has been found, the client still expresses the belief that there is a serious illness. These symptoms are typical of which of the following disorders?

    A. Conversion disorder
    B. Depersonalization
    C. Hypochondriasis
    D. Somatization disorder

16. A nurse is teaching a group of clients on substance abuse. A client asks what substance abuse is. The **best** response by the nurse is which of the following?

    A. An excessive drug use inconsistent with advised medical purposes
    B. A physiological need for a drug
    C. A psychological dependence on a drug
    D. A compulsion to take a drug on either a continual or periodic basis

17. Which of the following is **most** reflective of a cognitive disorder?

    A. Suicidal thoughts
    B. Hallucination
    C. Feeling of dread
    D. Deficit in memory

18. A client begins to repeat phrases that others have just said. This type of speech is known as:

    A. Autism
    B. Neologism
    C. Echopraxia
    D. Echolalia

19. Which of the following would be the **best** example of a primary prevention designed as part of a community health outreach program.

    A. Stress prevention group
    B. Diabetes management group
    C. Anger management group
    D. HIV screening program

20. The nurse is caring for a client recently treated for a diagnosis of esophageal varices. Which is the **most** important information for the nurse to include in the teaching plan for the client?

    A. Decrease fluids to decrease congestive heart failure
    B. Avoid exercise to decrease bleeding
    C. Avoid straining during defecation to keep venous pressure low
    D. Decrease the amount of food consumed

Mark your answers in the book and enter the answer into your virtual trainer. The answers will be there. After each question mark whether you got it correct or not.  You must get a 95% on this exam

# CONGRATULATIONS – YOU'VE COMPLETED THE NCLEX VIRTUAL TRAINER!

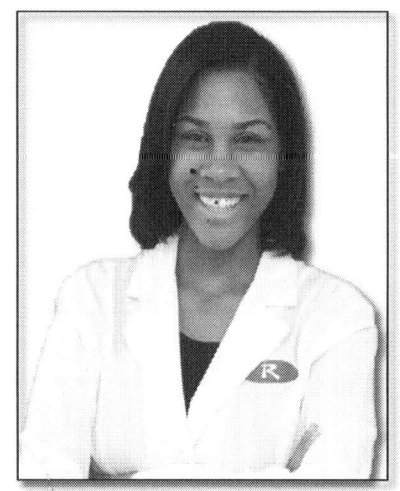

You're one step closer to sitting for NCLEX! As I said in the introduction to this book, I'm confident that if you haven't studied the content and honored the process that you can pass NCLEX!

Even if you are feeling a bit anxious I promise you it's normal! This test is important and I know that you can do it – in fact I want to see your testimonial video on the other side of NCLEX where you're smiling or sharing tears of joy as soon as you see your name on the board results and it has that big RN attached to it. You deserve that moment and just know that your success will not only bless you but it's going to bless everyone around you as well.

## BEFORE YOU TEST

After completing this resource you should know exactly what your next steps are for NCLEX. There are typically three options and remember you should always consider moving your test date back a few weeks whenever you need to finish studying the content. Don't allow a rush to test take you off of your A-Game! Your license is waiting on you but you have to be prepared in order to receive it!

1. **You're ready to test!** (How awesome is that you may just be days away from getting your license!)
2. **You may need to extend your VT access** in order to go back and review your weak areas before sitting for NCLEX! Which is a good thing especially as a repeat tester or foreign nurse
3. **You may want to do added questions** from the newly released **ReMar Nurse Virtual Question Bank!**

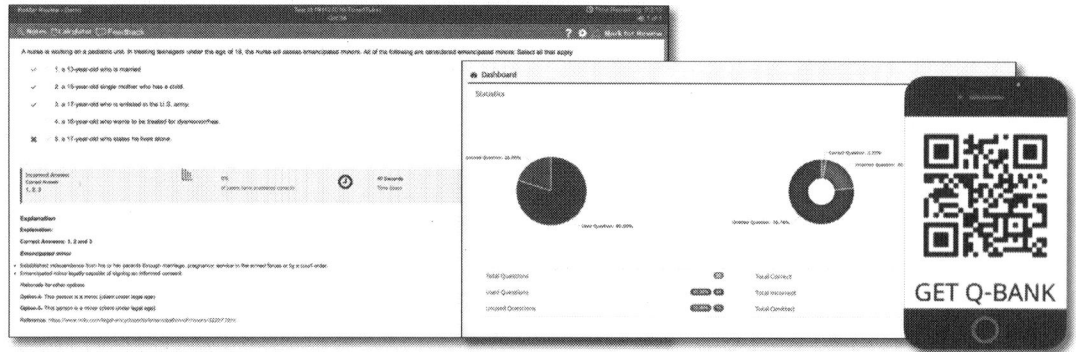

For more information or help selecting the best program please feel free to chat with our NCLEX experts at www.ReMarNurse.com or call 1-855-625-3966.